HOW TO DRAW ANATOMY

HOW TO DRAW ANATOMY

Phillip Molloy

ST4 Anaesthetic Registrar, The Grange University Hospital

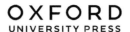

OXFORD
UNIVERSITY PRESS

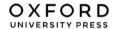

Great Clarendon Street, Oxford, OX2 6DP,
United Kingdom

Oxford University Press is a department of the University of Oxford.
It furthers the University's objective of excellence in research, scholarship,
and education by publishing worldwide. Oxford is a registered trade mark of
Oxford University Press in the UK and in certain other countries

Published in the United States of America by Oxford University Press
198 Madison Avenue, New York, NY 10016, United States of America

British Library Cataloguing in Publication Data

Data available

Library of Congress Control Number: 2022952182

ISBN 978–0–19–288332–2

DOI: 10.1093/med/9780192883322.001.0001

Printed and bound by
CPI Group (UK) Ltd, Croydon, CR0 4YY

Dedicated in memory of Earnie and Chita Harris.

FOREWORD

Prof Robert Kirby MD FRCS

Professor of Clinical Education and Surgery, Consultant Surgeon, and Dean of University Hospital of North Midlands

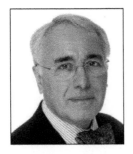

I applaud Dr Phill Molloy's work in producing this book. When I was working towards my primary fellowship exam in 1978, I learnt to draw and annotate anatomical diagrams. It was many years later that I helped Phill learn anatomy in the dissecting room!

Knowledge of anatomy is important for all doctors and others dealing with patients. It is, of course, vital for surgeons or other practitioners dealing directly with patients' bodies on a day-to-day basis to understand the intricacies of the parts they are working with.

The greatest advances in medical knowledge in the sixteenth century coincided with the learning of human anatomy after a thousand years of comparative ignorance, based on knowledge of animals rather than humans. Understanding the structure of the human body enabled the scientific minds of the late Middle Ages to work out much of its function and the workings. The most beautiful anatomical drawings were produced for a wider public by Vesalius and for a more limited audience by Leonardo da Vinci after their experiences of dissection. Anatomical textbooks since then have disseminated knowledge to generations of professionals.

This book teaches the learner to learn and remember basic anatomy by the application of drawing. Learning how to draw anatomical structures will assist with day-to-day understanding of anatomy and help students—both undergraduate and postgraduate—revise for anatomy exams.

I hope that this book proves popular and that it helps many people understand and remember anatomy and also pass their exams.

PREFACE

Dr Phill Molloy MBChB BSc (Hons) PGCert

ST4 Anaesthetic Registrar, The Grange University Hospital

Prior to the creation of this book, I found learning anatomy incredibly difficult. Looking at complicated and intricate textbook diagrams and then applying that knowledge in real life can be cumbersome, whether it be in the dissection room, operating theatre, or during exams.

This book will enable readers to both accurately reproduce anatomical drawings while also offering a template to appreciate variance in clinical practice. It also provides a comprehensive overview of anatomy for medical students and other healthcare professionals alike. Furthermore, these simple but concise illustrations may be kept as a toolkit to enhance explanations for patients visually during consultations without the need for expensive three-dimensional models—something that your patients will love (whether in clinical practice or during your OSCEs!).

The book has been designed with plenty of white space to allow the addition of notes during either anatomy classes or private study. I hope you enjoy this resource and welcome feedback or suggestions!

ACKNOWLEDGEMENTS

I would like to express my gratitude to the following individuals for their kind support, teaching, and help which have ultimately led to the production of this book.

To Professor Ruth Chambers OBE for mentoring me throughout the years as student and doctor, instilling the belief and discipline that almost anything can be achieved.

To Mr Joe Borucki, Dr Taha Haq, and Captain Jake Melhuish for their critical appraisals and moral support throughout.

To the student reviewers for your input and feedback.

To Keele University Medical School for its modern and ever-adapting and creative curriculum.

CONTENTS

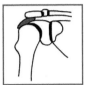

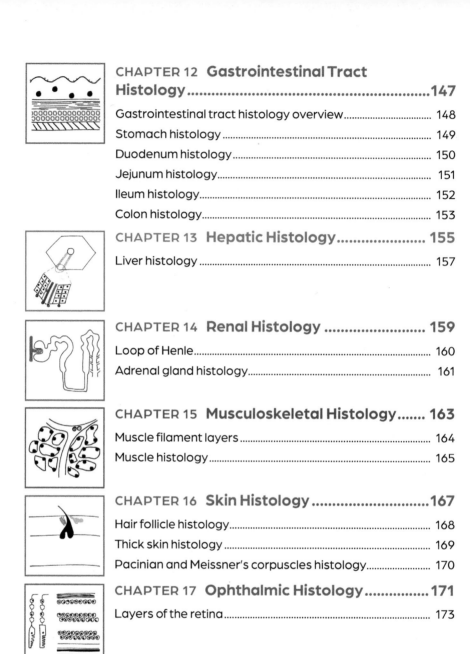

SENIOR REVIEWERS

JUNIOR REVIEWERS

Rahul Anil Bhagwat iBSc (Hons)
Year 4 Medical Student
University College London

Georgia Brown
Year 3 Medical Student
University of Newcastle (Australia)

Max Butler
Year 3 Medical Student
University of Cambridge

Kaylise Faull
Year 4 Medical Student
University of Newcastle (Australia)

Simon Hickey
Year 3 Medical Student
University of Newcastle (Australia)

Akos Marton
Year 3 Medical Student
University of Cambridge

Michael McLucas
Year 4 Medical Student
University of Newcastle (Australia)

Maria Elaine Prayle BSc (Hons)
Year 3 Medical Student
University of Keele

Emily Wales BSc (Hons)
Year 3 Medical Student
Cardiff University

Ben Walters
Year 4 Medical Student
University of Keele

Jack FG Wellington
Year 3 Medical Student
Cardiff University

Jessica Xie BSc (Hons)
Year 4 Medical Student
University College London

HOW TO ... USE THE BOOK

Learn How To Draw, Then How To Label!

- Follow the diagrams in number order.
- Each consecutive diagram has additional features to add on.
- Once complete, use the larger drawing (diagram usually on the next page) to learn structures and diagram labelling.
- Finally, test yourself and your friends!

How To ... Orientate

- Crosshatches (or compasses) are useful for determining your orientation.
- Whenever drawing, always remember to include one! It will help you determine your orientation for labelling—particularly in exams.
- It allows you to orientate the diagram in two dimensions.
- Note below how the second crosshatch shows 'L' (left) to be on the right side and 'R' (right) to be on the left side (as you look at it). Just as you would interpret a chest radiograph depending whether you are looking at the image from the front (anterior to posterior) or back (posterior to anterior), left or right may be on one side or the other.

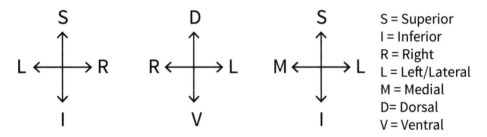

S = Superior
I = Inferior
R = Right
L = Left/Lateral
M = Medial
D= Dorsal
V = Ventral

Lines Key

———————— Solid blue line: structure running anteriorly

— — — — Fenestrated blue line: structure running posteriorly

CHAPTER ONE

CARDIOVASCULAR

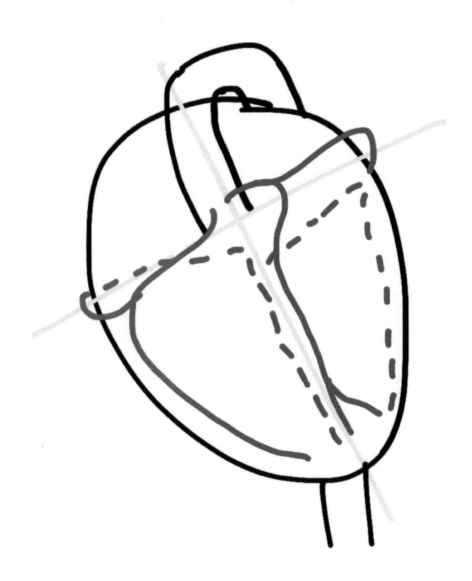

HOW TO ... DRAW THE MAJOR CARDIAC VESSELS

1)

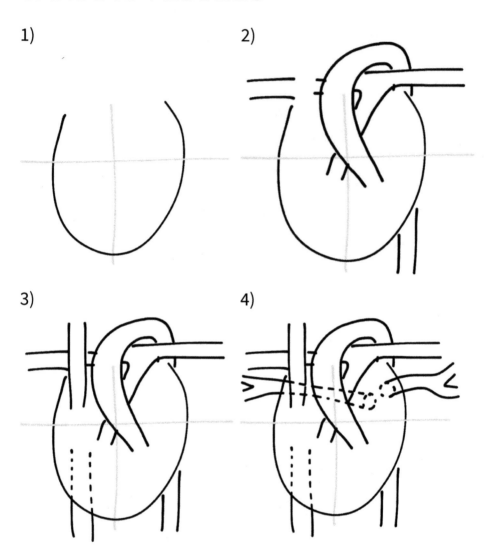

2)

3)

4)

THE MAJOR CARDIAC VESSELS

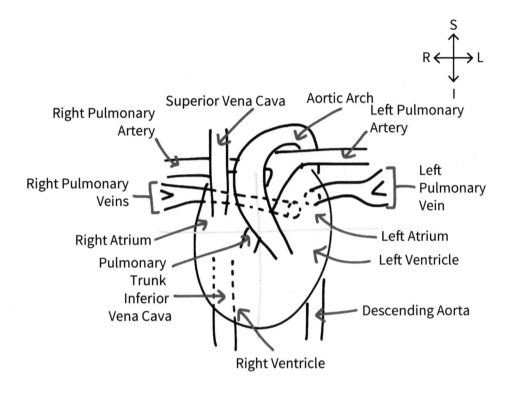

S
R ← → **L**
I

Right Pulmonary Artery

Superior Vena Cava

Aortic Arch

Left Pulmonary Artery

Right Pulmonary Veins

Left Pulmonary Vein

Right Atrium

Left Atrium

Pulmonary Trunk

Left Ventricle

Inferior Vena Cava

Descending Aorta

Right Ventricle

🔥 **HOT TIPS**

NB: The Aorta runs posterior to the heart (not fully shown in this image to give greater clarity).

HOW TO … DRAW THE 1ST BRANCHES OF THE AORTA

1)

2)

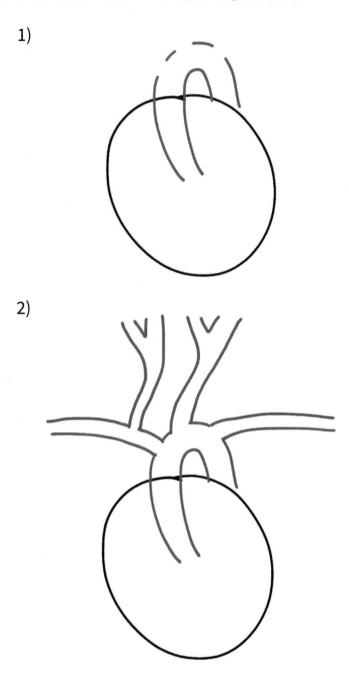

THE 1ST BRANCHES OF THE AORTA

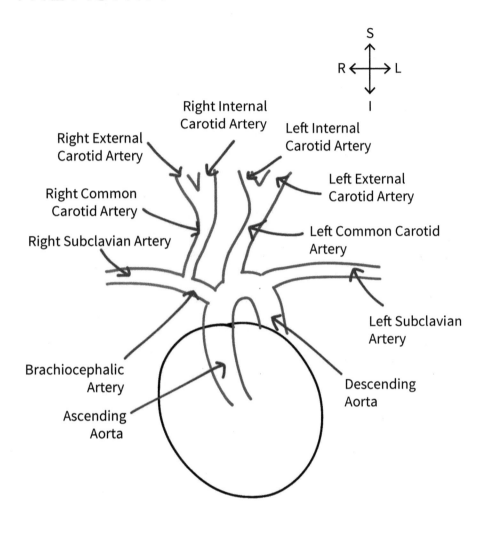

S

R ← → L

I

Right Internal Carotid Artery

Right External Carotid Artery

Left Internal Carotid Artery

Right Common Carotid Artery

Left External Carotid Artery

Right Subclavian Artery

Left Common Carotid Artery

Left Subclavian Artery

Brachiocephalic Artery

Descending Aorta

Ascending Aorta

HOW TO … DRAW THE GREAT VEINS

1)

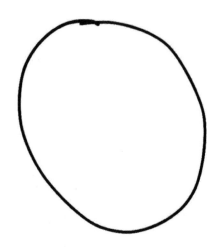

2)

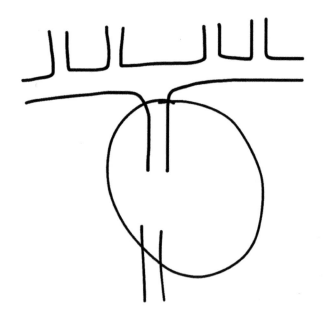

THE GREAT VEINS

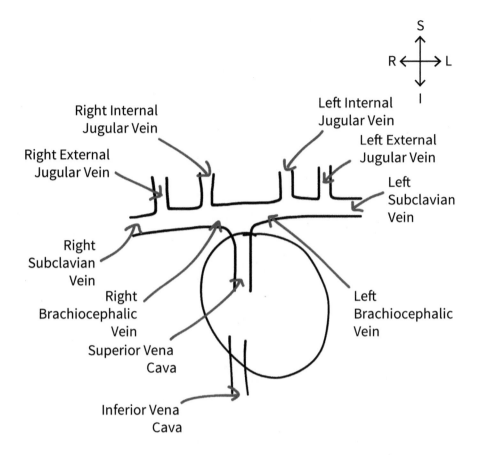

S

R ←→ L

I

Right Internal
Jugular Vein

Left Internal
Jugular Vein

Left External
Jugular Vein

Right External
Jugular Vein

Left
Subclavian
Vein

Right
Subclavian
Vein

Right
Brachiocephalic
Vein

Left
Brachiocephalic
Vein

Superior Vena
Cava

Inferior Vena
Cava

HOW TO ... DRAW THE CARDIAC VALVES

1)

2)

3)

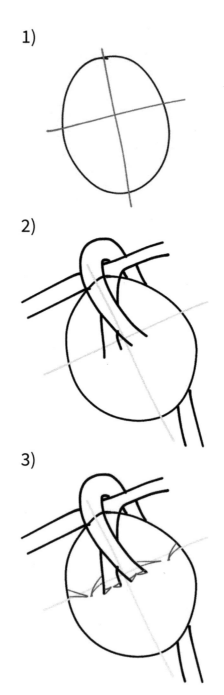

THE CARDIAC VALVES

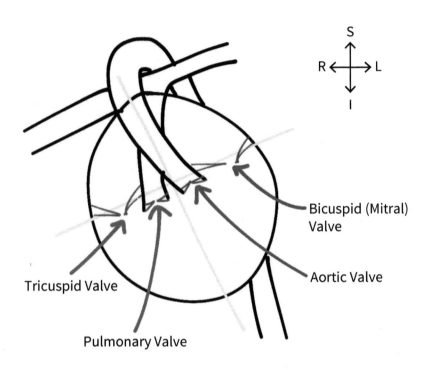

S
R ← → L
I

Bicuspid (Mitral) Valve

Aortic Valve

Tricuspid Valve

Pulmonary Valve

🔥 **HOT TIPS** **Valve structure**

Tricuspid has three leaflets.

Bicuspid has two leaflets ('Mitral' is derived from mitre—a bishop's two-pointed hat).

HOW TO ... DRAW THE CORONARY ARTERIES

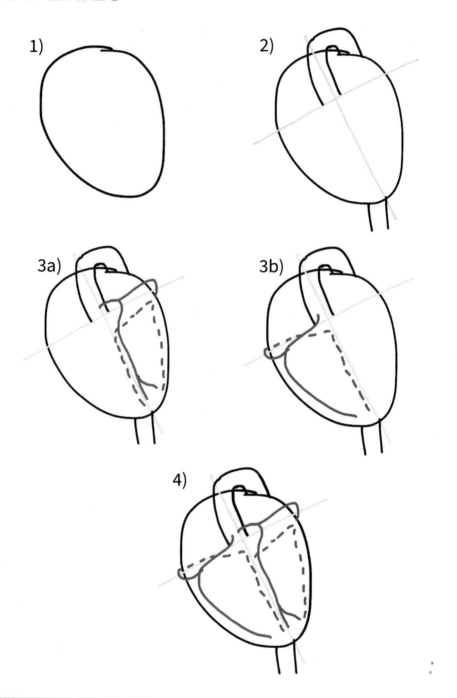

1)

2)

3a)

3b)

4)

THE CORONARY ARTERIES (ANTERIOR VIEW)

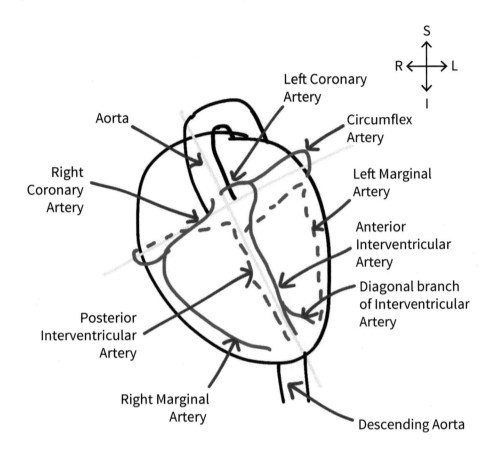

Left Coronary Artery

Aorta

Circumflex Artery

Right Coronary Artery

Left Marginal Artery

Anterior Interventricular Artery

Diagonal branch of Interventricular Artery

Posterior Interventricular Artery

Right Marginal Artery

Descending Aorta

S
R ← → L
I

 HOT TIPS

NB: the Anterior Interventricular Artery is also known as the Left Anterior Descending (LAD).

HOW TO ... DRAW THE CORONARY VEINS

1)

2)

3a)

3b)

4)

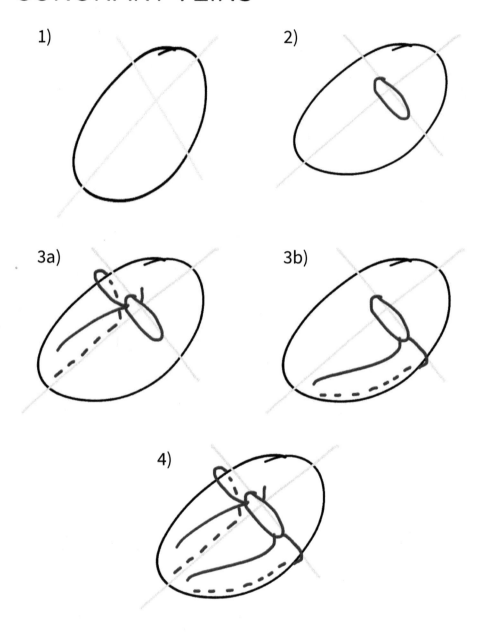

THE CORONARY VEINS (POSTERIOR VIEW)

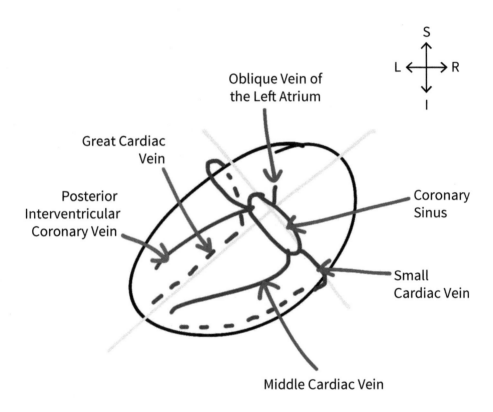

Oblique Vein of the Left Atrium

Great Cardiac Vein

Posterior Interventricular Coronary Vein

Coronary Sinus

Small Cardiac Vein

Middle Cardiac Vein

S
L R
I

CHAPTER TWO

RESPIRATORY

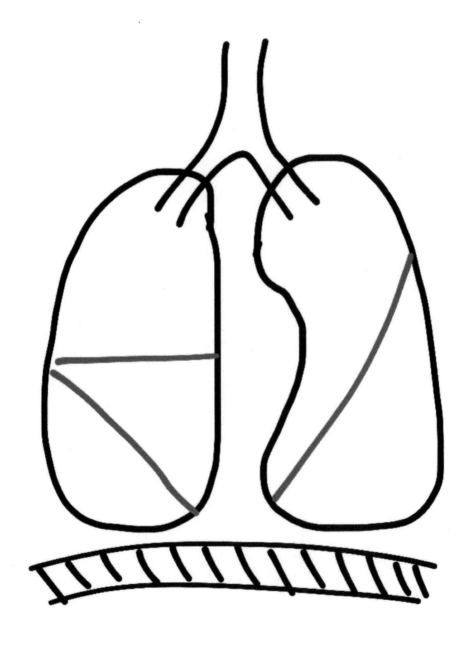

HOW TO ... DRAW THE LUNGS

1)

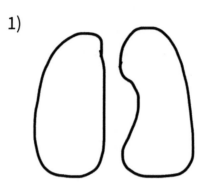

2)

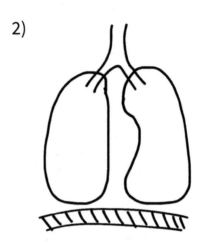

3)

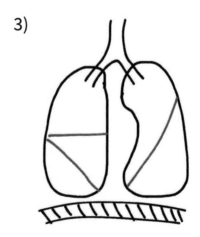

THE LUNGS

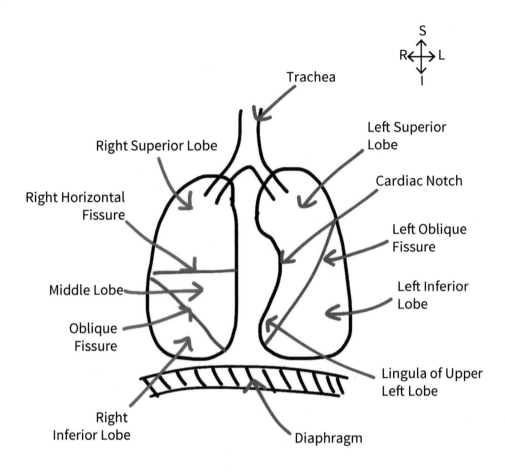

Trachea

S
R ← ✛ → L
I

Right Superior Lobe

Left Superior Lobe

Cardiac Notch

Right Horizontal Fissure

Left Oblique Fissure

Middle Lobe

Left Inferior Lobe

Oblique Fissure

Lingula of Upper Left Lobe

Right Inferior Lobe

Diaphragm

> 🔥 **HOT TIPS**
> Right Horizontal Fissure: follows the 4th rib.
> Right Oblique Fissure: follows the 6th rib.
> Left Oblique Fissure: follows the 6th rib.

HOW TO … DRAW THE TRACHEA

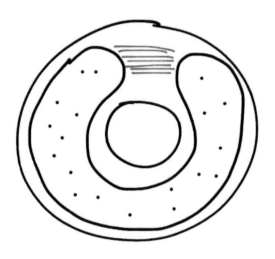

CROSS SECTION OF THE TRACHEA

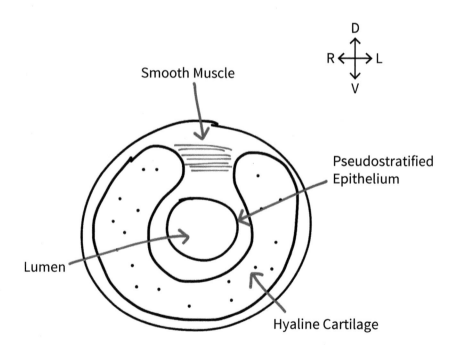

Smooth Muscle

D
R ←→ L
V

Pseudostratified
Epithelium

Lumen

Hyaline Cartilage

DRAW A CROSS SECTION OF THE BRONCHUS

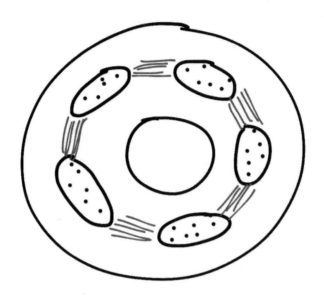

CROSS SECTION OF THE BRONCHUS

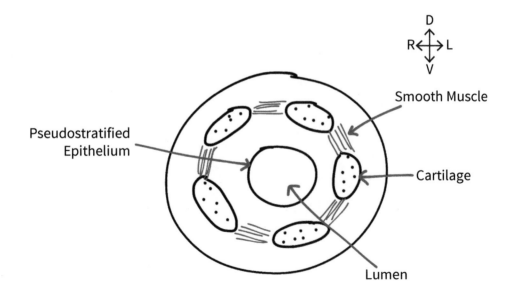

Pseudostratified Epithelium

Smooth Muscle

Cartilage

Lumen

HOW TO ... DRAW CROSS SECTION OF THE BRONCHIOLE

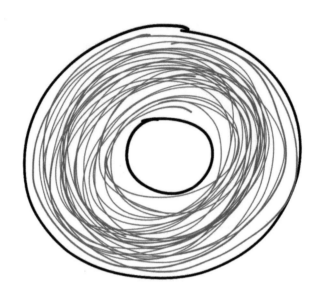

CROSS SECTION OF THE BRONCHIOLE

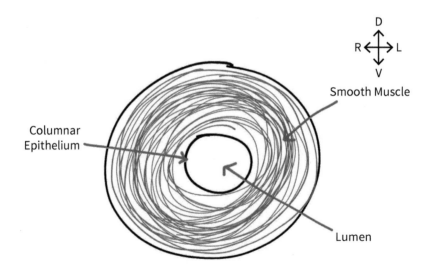

D

R ↔ L

V

Smooth Muscle

Columnar
Epithelium

Lumen

HOW TO ... DRAW THE THORACIC LAYERS

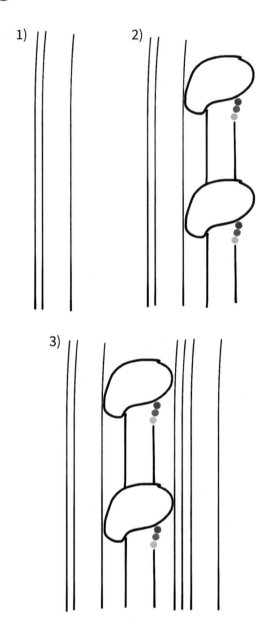

1)

2)

3)

THE THORACIC LAYERS

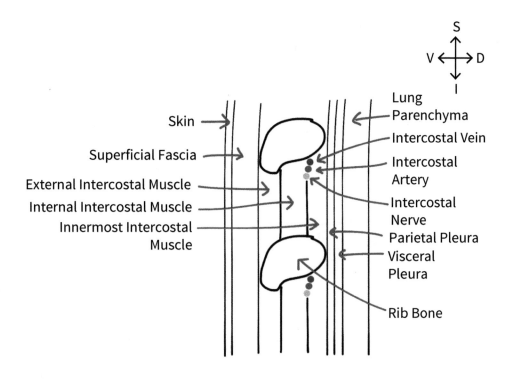

S

V ←→ D

I

Skin →

Superficial Fascia →

External Intercostal Muscle →

Internal Intercostal Muscle →

Innermost Intercostal Muscle →

Lung Parenchyma ←

Intercostal Vein

Intercostal Artery

Intercostal Nerve

Parietal Pleura ←

Visceral Pleura ←

Rib Bone

🔥 **HOT TIPS**

Remember VAN for order of structures under the rib:

V = Vein

A = Artery

N = Nerve

NB: the neurovascular bundle sits between the Internal and Innermost Intercostal Muscles.

HOW TO ... DRAW THE RIB

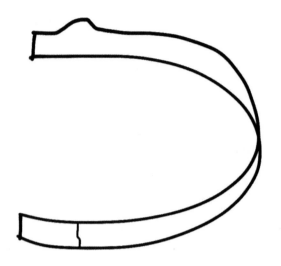

THE RIB

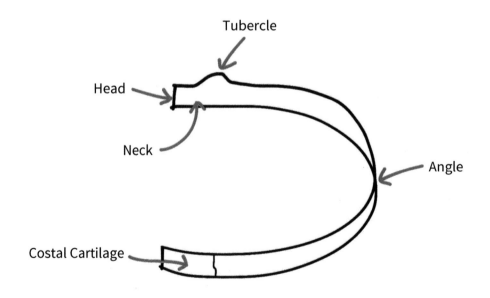

HOW TO ... DRAW VENOUS DRAINAGE OF THE THORAX

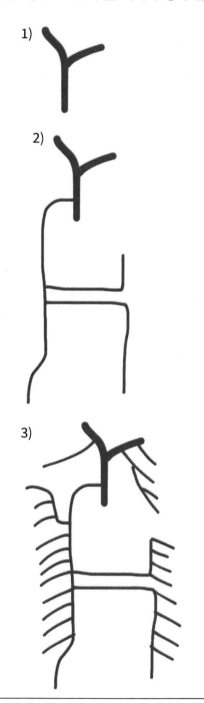

1)

2)

3)

VENOUS DRAINAGE OF THE THORAX

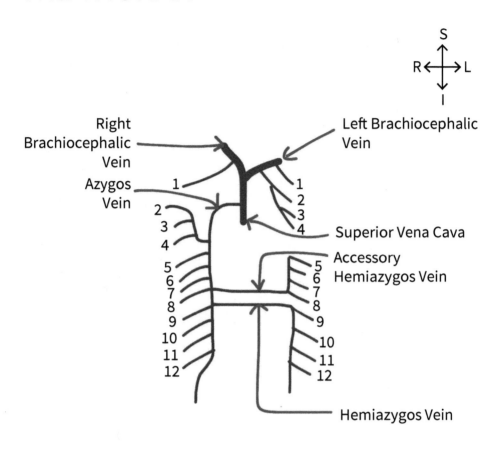

CHAPTER THREE

UPPER GASTROINTESTINAL

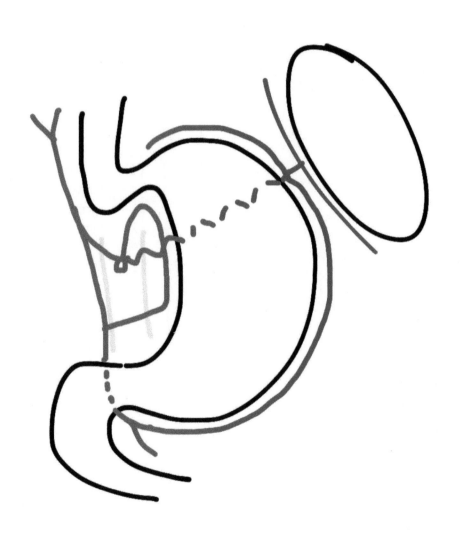

LAYERS OF THE ABDOMINAL WALL (LONGITUDINAL VIEW)

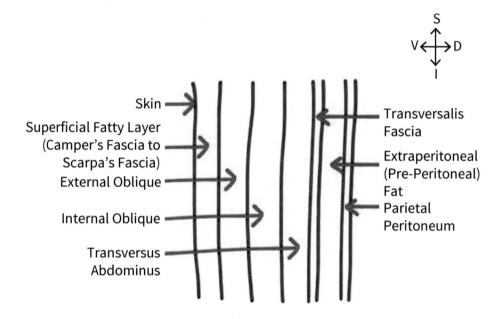

Skin

Superficial Fatty Layer (Camper's Fascia to Scarpa's Fascia)

External Oblique

Internal Oblique

Transversus Abdominus

Transversalis Fascia

Extraperitoneal (Pre-Peritoneal) Fat

Parietal Peritoneum

🔥 **HOT TIPS**

NB: Transversus Abdominus is also known as Endoabdominal Fascia.

ANATOMY OF THE STOMACH

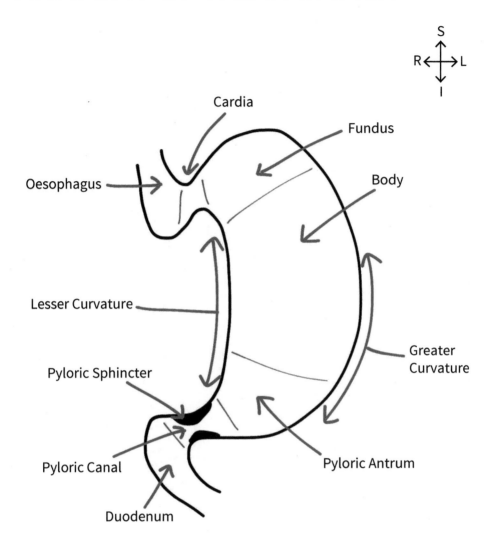

Cardia

Fundus

Oesophagus

Body

Lesser Curvature

Greater Curvature

Pyloric Sphincter

Pyloric Canal

Pyloric Antrum

Duodenum

S

R ← → L

I

HOW TO ... DRAW THE BLOOD SUPPLY TO THE STOMACH

1)

2)

3)

4)

5)

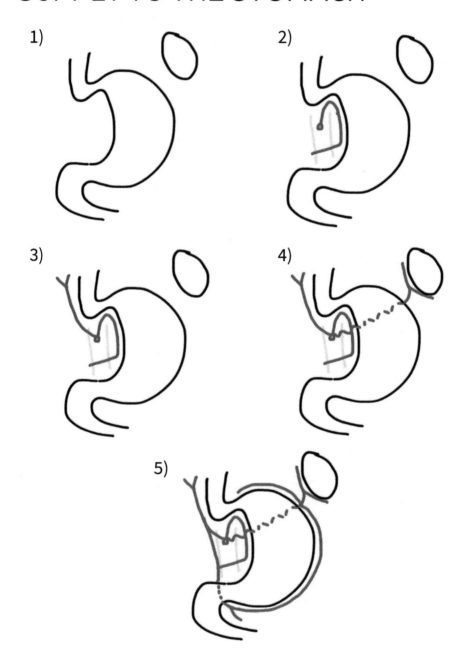

ARTERIAL BLOOD SUPPLY TO THE STOMACH

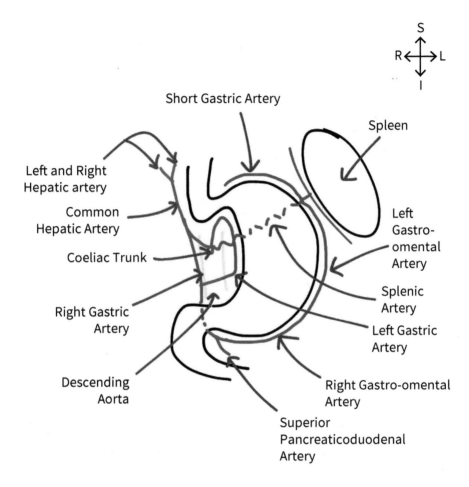

S

R ←→ L

I

Short Gastric Artery

Spleen

Left and Right Hepatic artery

Common Hepatic Artery

Coeliac Trunk

Left Gastro-omental Artery

Splenic Artery

Right Gastric Artery

Left Gastric Artery

Descending Aorta

Right Gastro-omental Artery

Superior Pancreaticoduodenal Artery

🔥 HOT TIPS Vertebral levels of aortic branches

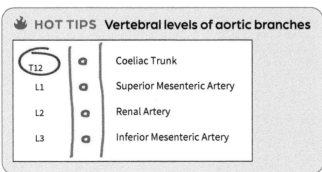

T12		Coeliac Trunk
L1		Superior Mesenteric Artery
L2		Renal Artery
L3		Inferior Mesenteric Artery

CHAPTER FOUR
LOWER GASTROINTESTINAL

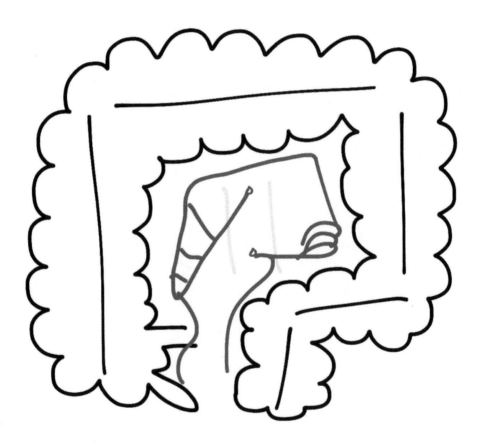

THE LARGE INTESTINE

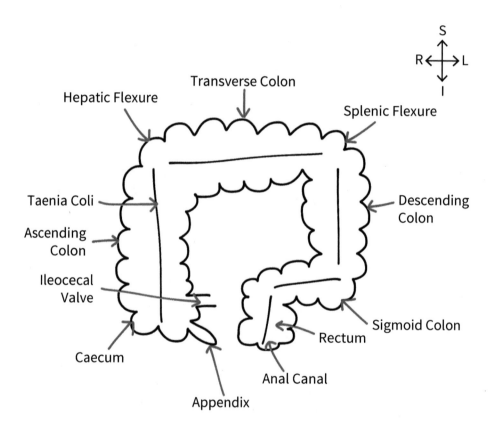

Transverse Colon

Hepatic Flexure

Splenic Flexure

Taenia Coli

Descending Colon

Ascending Colon

Ileocecal Valve

Sigmoid Colon

Caecum

Rectum

Anal Canal

Appendix

S

R

L

I

HOW TO ... DRAW THE BLOOD SUPPLY TO THE LARGE INTESTINE

1)

2)

3)

4)

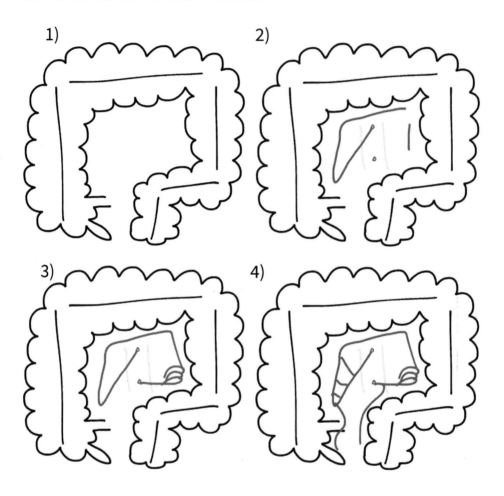

ARTERIAL BLOOD SUPPLY TO THE LARGE INTESTINE

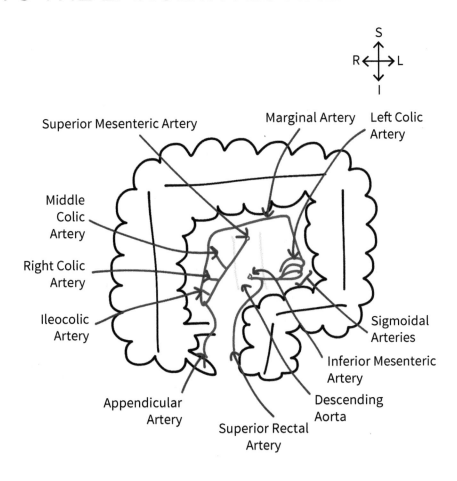

S
R ← → L
I

Superior Mesenteric Artery

Marginal Artery

Left Colic Artery

Middle Colic Artery

Right Colic Artery

Ileocolic Artery

Appendicular Artery

Superior Rectal Artery

Sigmoidal Arteries

Inferior Mesenteric Artery

Descending Aorta

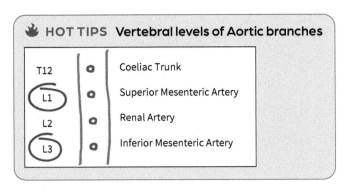

🔥 **HOT TIPS** **Vertebral levels of Aortic branches**

T12	▫	Coeliac Trunk
L1	▫	Superior Mesenteric Artery
L2	▫	Renal Artery
L3	▫	Inferior Mesenteric Artery

CHAPTER FIVE

HEPATOBILIARY

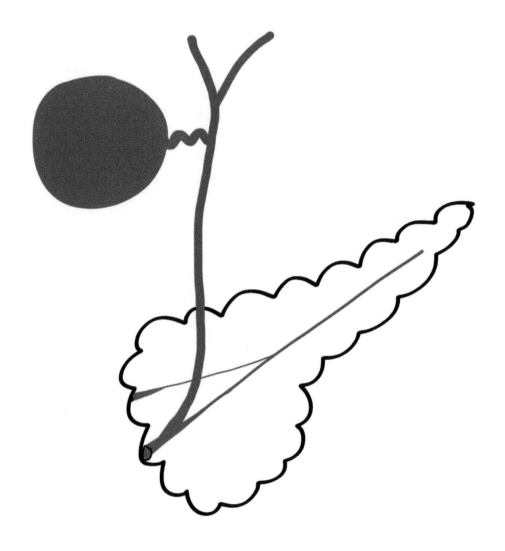

HOW TO ... DRAW THE PANCREAS

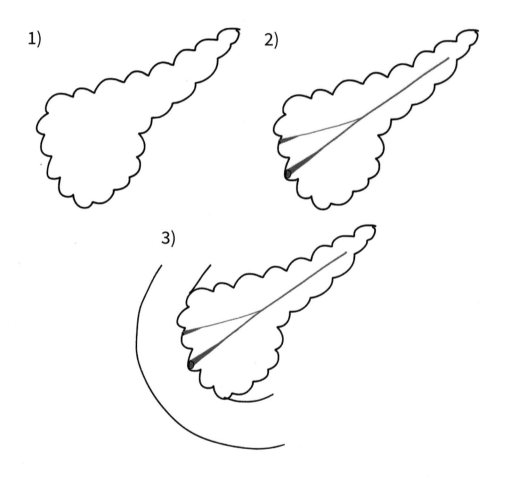

1)

2)

3)

THE PANCREAS

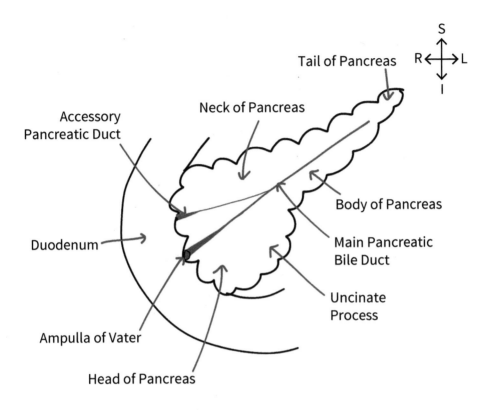

Tail of Pancreas

S
R ← → L
I

Neck of Pancreas

Accessory
Pancreatic Duct

Body of Pancreas

Duodenum

Main Pancreatic
Bile Duct

Uncinate
Process

Ampulla of Vater

Head of Pancreas

🔥 HOT TIPS

The Accessory Pancreatic Duct comes off the Main Pancreatic Duct.

Bile and pancreatic enzymes meet at the Ampulla of Vater.

NB: the Main Pancreatic Duct does **NOT** contain bile. It contains pancreatic enzymes!

HOW TO ... DRAW ANATOMY OF THE BILIARY TREE

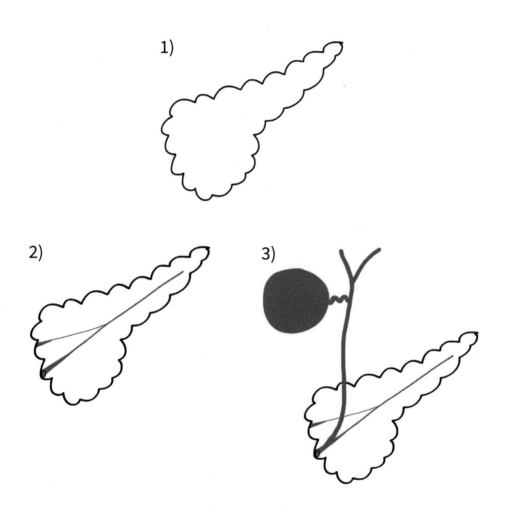

1)

2)

3)

THE BILIARY TREE

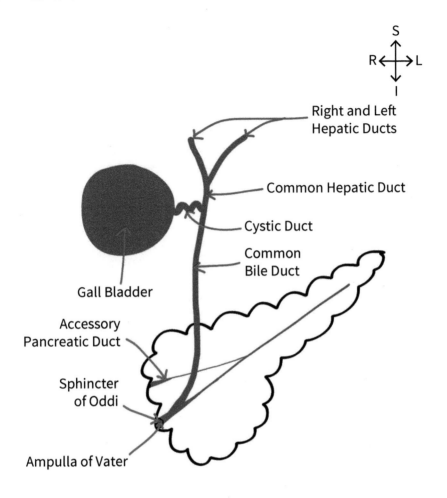

S
R ←→ L
I

Right and Left Hepatic Ducts

Common Hepatic Duct

Cystic Duct

Common Bile Duct

Gall Bladder

Accessory Pancreatic Duct

Sphincter of Oddi

Ampulla of Vater

🔥 **HOT TIPS**

The Ampulla of Vater is formed by the union of the Pancreatic Duct and the Common Bile Duct.

The Sphincter of Oddi controls the flow of pancreatic and bile juices through the Ampulla of Vater.

HOW TO ... DRAW THE BILIARY TREE AND SURROUNDING ORGANS

1)

2)

3)

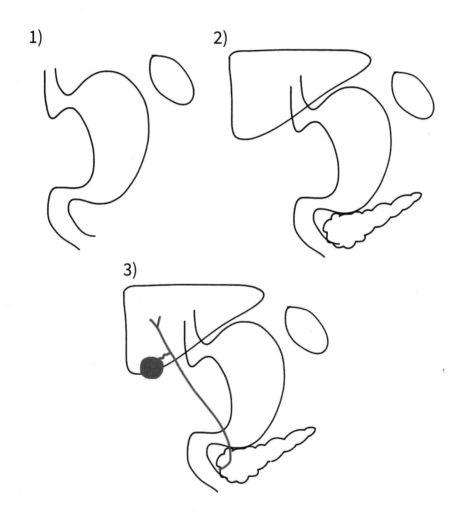

THE BILIARY TREE AND SURROUNDING ORGANS

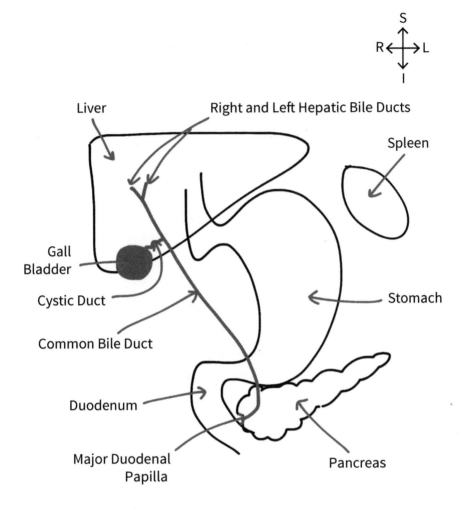

S
R ← → L
I

Liver

Right and Left Hepatic Bile Ducts

Spleen

Gall Bladder

Cystic Duct

Stomach

Common Bile Duct

Duodenum

Major Duodenal Papilla

Pancreas

HOW TO ... DRAW ANTERIOR VIEW OF THE LIVER

1)

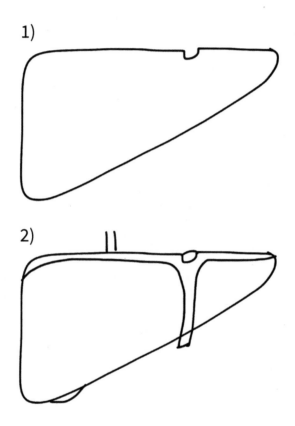

2)

ANTERIOR VIEW OF THE LIVER

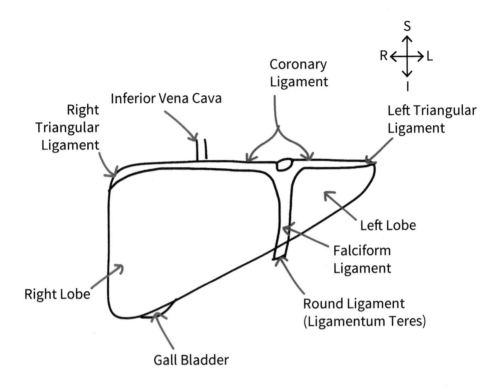

S
R ← → L
I

Coronary Ligament

Inferior Vena Cava

Right Triangular Ligament

Left Triangular Ligament

Left Lobe

Falciform Ligament

Right Lobe

Round Ligament (Ligamentum Teres)

Gall Bladder

 HOT TIPS
The Round Ligament is also known as the Ligamentum Teres.

HOW TO ... DRAW POSTERIOR VIEW OF THE LIVER

1)

2)

3)

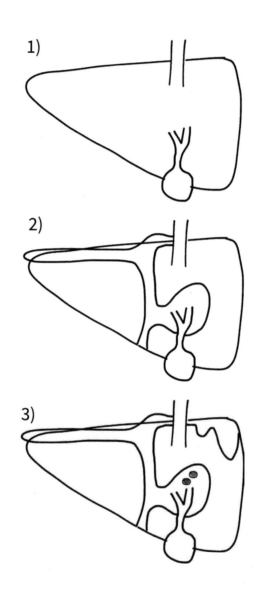

POSTERIOR VIEW OF THE LIVER

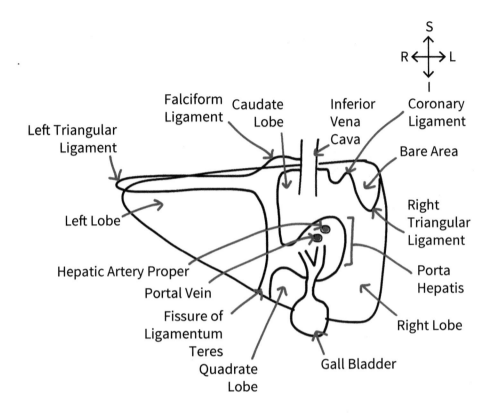

S
R ← → L
I

Falciform Ligament

Caudate Lobe

Inferior Vena Cava

Coronary Ligament

Left Triangular Ligament

Bare Area

Left Lobe

Right Triangular Ligament

Hepatic Artery Proper

Portal Vein

Porta Hepatis

Fissure of Ligamentum Teres

Right Lobe

Quadrate Lobe

Gall Bladder

🔥 **HOT TIPS**

How to remember which lobe is the Caudate or Quadrate?

1) The Gall Bladder looks like the letter Q—therefore think Quadrate Lobe.
2) The Caudate Lobe is next to the Inferior Vena Cava.

NB: The Common Hepatic Duct doesn't split into two until it's inside the liver (unlike it is shown here).

HOW TO ... DRAW INFERIOR VIEW OF THE LIVER

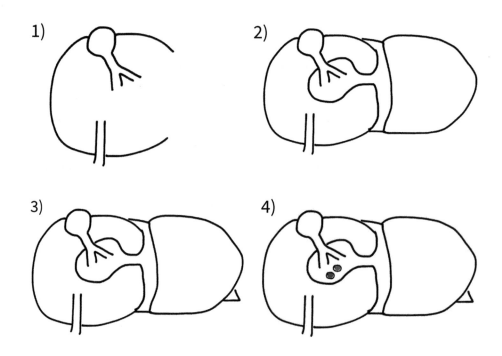

1)

2)

3)

4)

INFERIOR VIEW OF THE LIVER

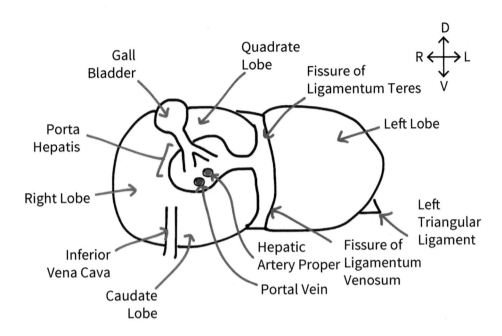

Gall Bladder

Quadrate Lobe

Fissure of Ligamentum Teres

D
R ← → L
V

Left Lobe

Porta Hepatis

Right Lobe

Left Triangular Ligament

Inferior Vena Cava

Hepatic Artery Proper

Fissure of Ligamentum Venosum

Portal Vein

Caudate Lobe

🔥 HOT TIPS

It looks like a bird!

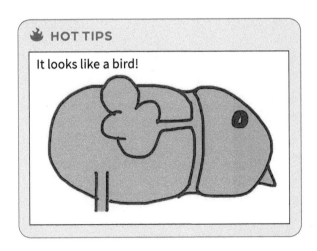

VENOUS DRAINAGE OF THE LIVER

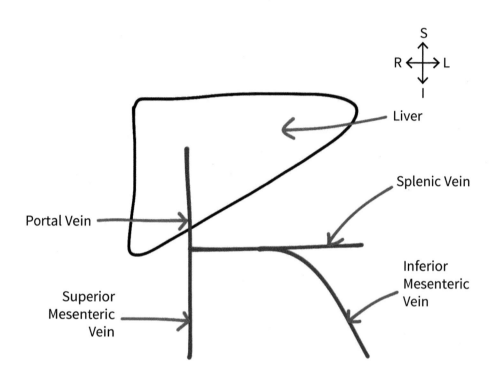

Liver

Splenic Vein

Inferior Mesenteric Vein

Portal Vein

Superior Mesenteric Vein

🔥 **HOT TIPS**
It is in the shape of the letter K (the Liver stores vitamin K).

CHAPTER SIX

NEUROLOGY

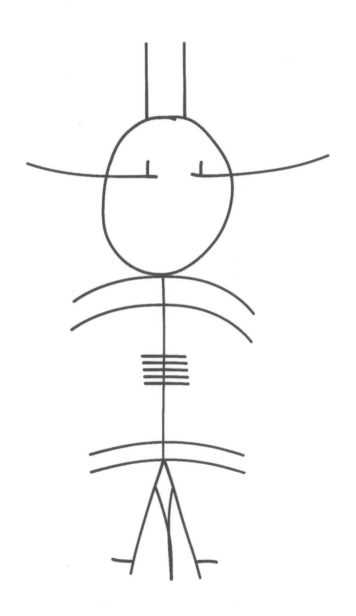

HOW TO ... DRAW THE LOBES OF THE BRAIN

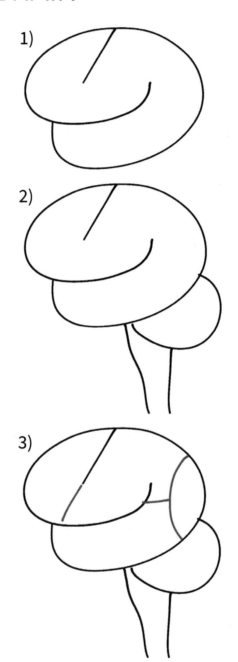

1)

2)

3)

LOBES OF THE BRAIN

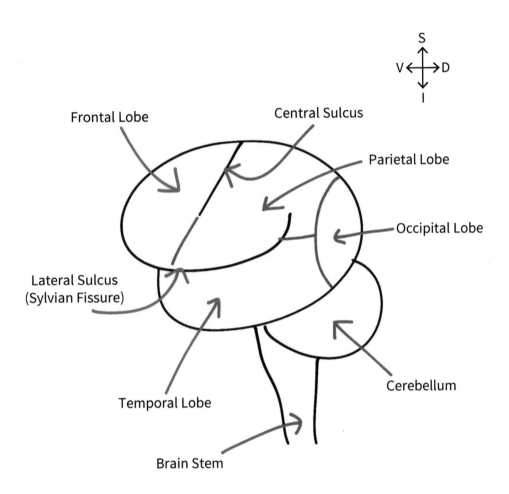

Frontal Lobe

Central Sulcus

Parietal Lobe

Occipital Lobe

Lateral Sulcus
(Sylvian Fissure)

Cerebellum

Temporal Lobe

Brain Stem

S

V ← → D

I

THE DURA

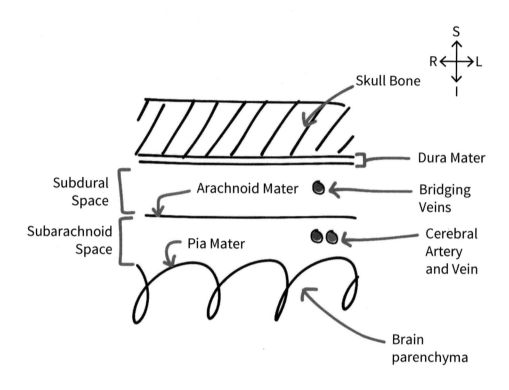

Skull Bone

Dura Mater

Subdural Space

Arachnoid Mater

Bridging Veins

Subarachnoid Space

Pia Mater

Cerebral Artery and Vein

Brain parenchyma

🔥 **HOT TIPS**

The Dura Mater has two layers which are usually in continuum (periosteal periosteum in contact with the skull and meningeal meninges inferior to this). They only split apart to form venous sinuses. The extradural space is the area between the dura and the skull. Cerebrospinal fluid flows within the subarachnoid space.

HOW TO … DRAW CROSS SECTION OF THE SPINAL CORD

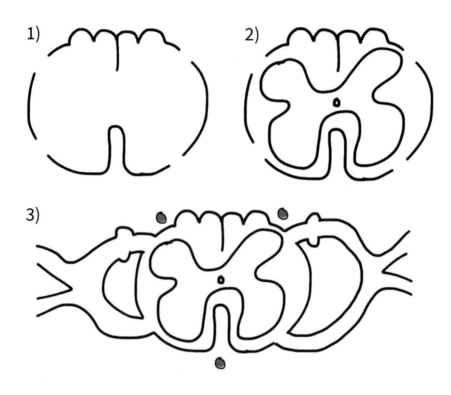

1)

2)

3)

CROSS SECTION OF THE SPINAL CORD

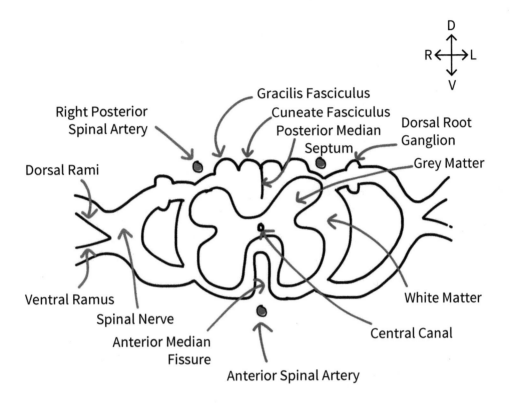

D

R ← → L

V

Gracilis Fasciculus

Cuneate Fasciculus

Right Posterior Spinal Artery

Posterior Median Septum

Dorsal Root Ganglion

Dorsal Rami

Grey Matter

Ventral Ramus

Spinal Nerve

Anterior Median Fissure

Anterior Spinal Artery

White Matter

Central Canal

> 🔥 **HOT TIPS**
> The Gracilis Fasciculus and Cuneate Fasciculus together make up the Dorsal Column.

HOW TO ... DRAW THE SPINAL CORD NUCLEI

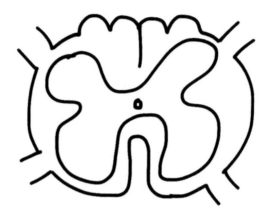

CROSS SECTIONAL VIEW OF SPINAL CORD NUCLEI

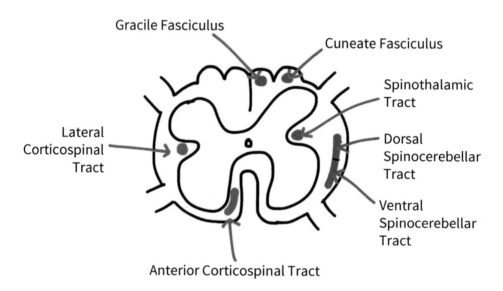

Gracile Fasciculus

Cuneate Fasciculus

Spinothalamic Tract

Lateral Corticospinal Tract

Dorsal Spinocerebellar Tract

Ventral Spinocerebellar Tract

Anterior Corticospinal Tract

HOW TO ... DRAW SPINAL TRACTS

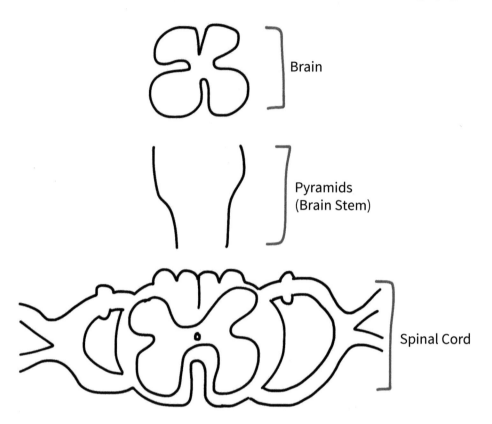

Brain

Pyramids
(Brain Stem)

Spinal Cord

 HOT TIPS
Use this basic template to practise your tract drawings.

SPINOTHALAMIC TRACT

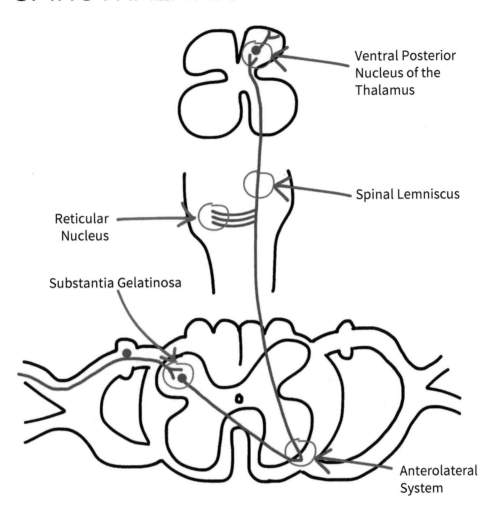

Ventral Posterior Nucleus of the Thalamus

Spinal Lemniscus

Reticular Nucleus

Substantia Gelatinosa

Anterolateral System

 HOT TIPS **Function (PICT)**
Pain.
Itch.
Crude touch and pressure.
Temperature.

DORSAL COLUMN TRACT

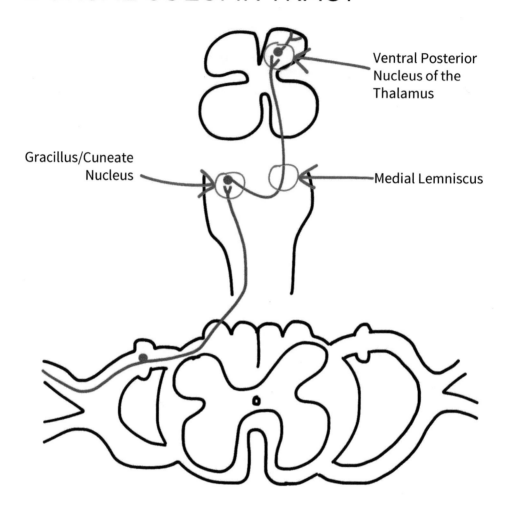

Ventral Posterior
Nucleus of the
Thalamus

Gracillus/Cuneate
Nucleus

Medial Lemniscus

 HOT TIPS Function (PDVF)
Proprioception.
Two touch Discrimination.
Vibration.
Fine touch.

CORTICOSPINAL TRACT

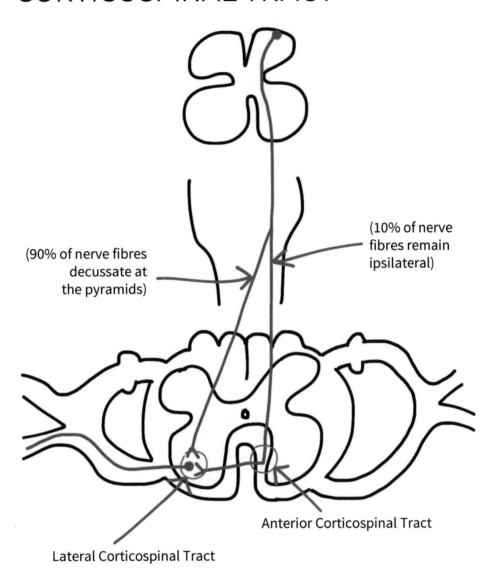

(90% of nerve fibres decussate at the pyramids)

(10% of nerve fibres remain ipsilateral)

Anterior Corticospinal Tract

Lateral Corticospinal Tract

🔥 HOT TIPS **Function (movement)**
Fine motor control.

HOW TO ... DRAW THE BRAIN STEM AND CRANIAL NERVES

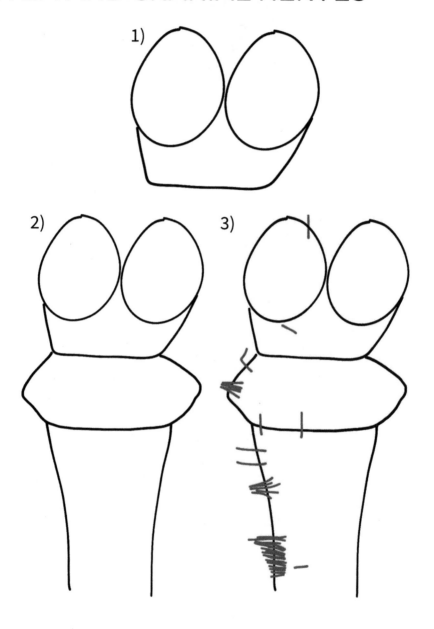

1)

2)

3)

THE BRAIN STEM AND CRANIAL NERVES

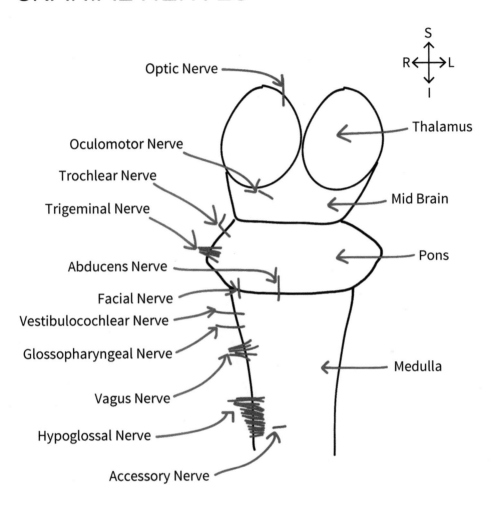

Optic Nerve

Thalamus

Oculomotor Nerve

Trochlear Nerve

Trigeminal Nerve

Mid Brain

Abducens Nerve

Pons

Facial Nerve

Vestibulocochlear Nerve

Glossopharyngeal Nerve

Medulla

Vagus Nerve

Hypoglossal Nerve

Accessory Nerve

🔥 HOT TIPS

Rule of thumb—list cranial nerves in order of their number except swap nerves 11 and 12.

The trochlear nerve is the only nerve to arise from the dorsal aspect of the brainstem.

HOW TO ... DRAW THE BASAL GANGLIA

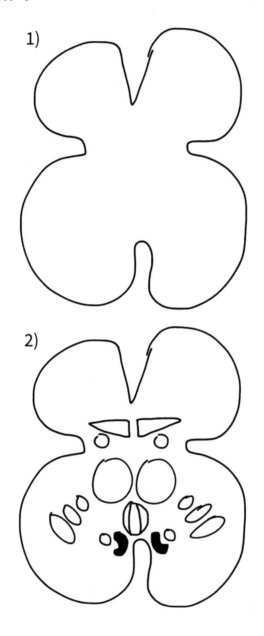

1)

2)

THE BASAL GANGLIA

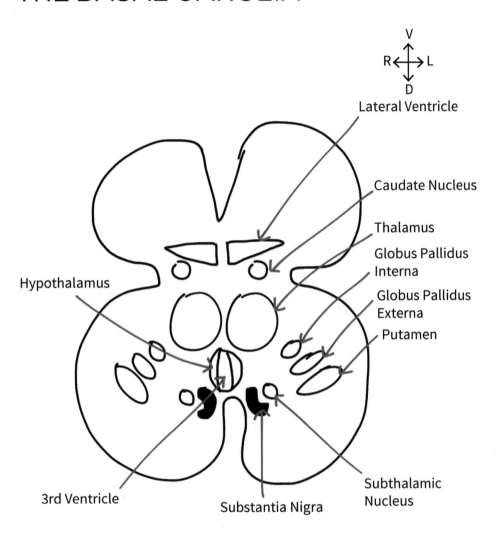

V

R ← → L

D

Lateral Ventricle

Caudate Nucleus

Thalamus

Globus Pallidus Interna

Globus Pallidus Externa

Putamen

Hypothalamus

Subthalamic Nucleus

3rd Ventricle

Substantia Nigra

🔥 HOT TIPS

Substantia Nigra is black (Nigra is Latin for black).

The Striatum is made up of the Putamen and Globus Pallidus Interna and Externa.

HOW TO ... DRAW THE VENTRICLES: LATERAL VIEW

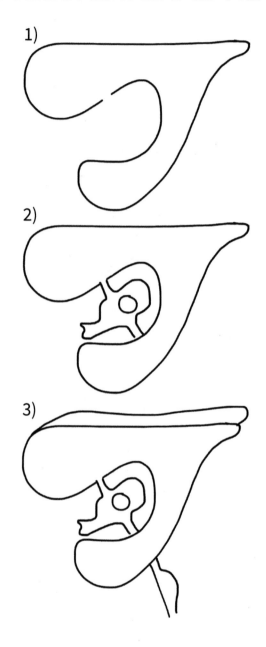

1)

2)

3)

THE VENTRICULAR SYSTEM: LATERAL VIEW

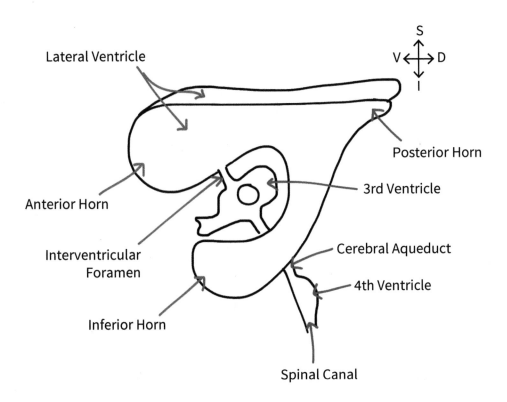

Lateral Ventricle

Posterior Horn

3rd Ventricle

Anterior Horn

Cerebral Aqueduct

Interventricular Foramen

4th Ventricle

Inferior Horn

Spinal Canal

S
V←→D
I

🔥 **HOT TIPS**
Lateral ventricles are the 1st and 2nd ventricles.

HOW TO ... DRAW THE VENTRICULAR SYSTEM: CORONAL VIEW

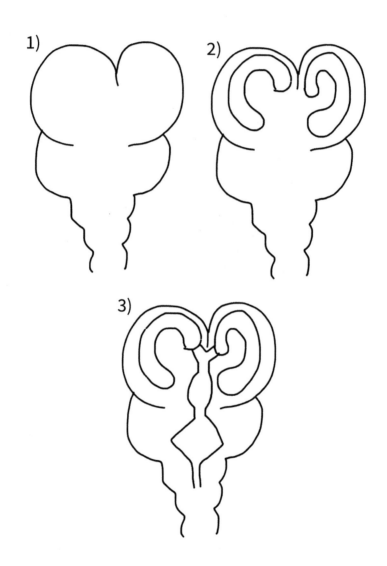

THE VENTRICULAR SYSTEM: CORONAL VIEW

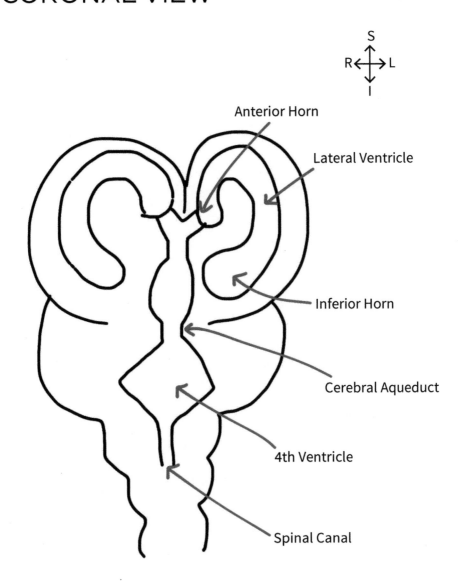

S

R ←→ L

I

Anterior Horn

Lateral Ventricle

Inferior Horn

Cerebral Aqueduct

4th Ventricle

Spinal Canal

HOW TO … DRAW THE CIRCLE OF WILLIS

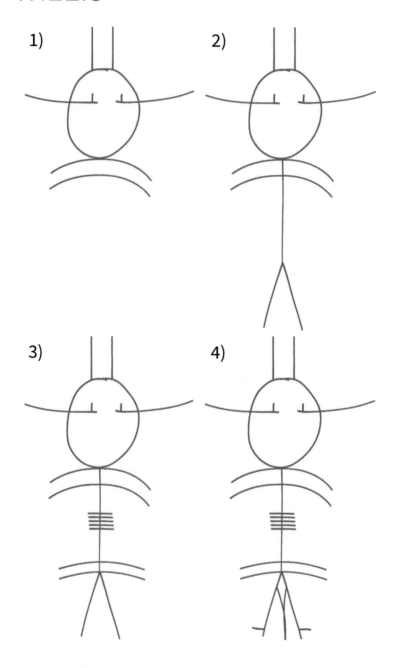

1)

2)

3)

4)

THE CIRCLE OF WILLIS

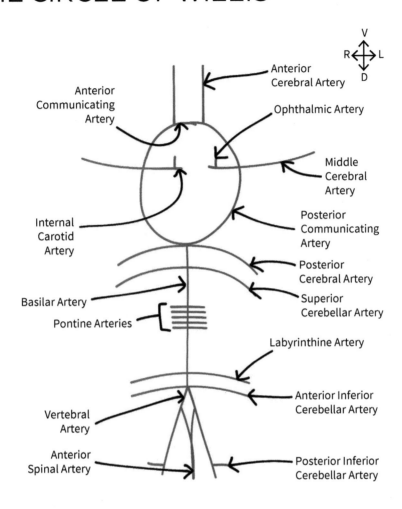

V
R ←+→ L
D

Anterior Cerebral Artery

Anterior Communicating Artery

Ophthalmic Artery

Middle Cerebral Artery

Internal Carotid Artery

Posterior Communicating Artery

Posterior Cerebral Artery

Basilar Artery

Superior Cerebellar Artery

Pontine Arteries

Labyrinthine Artery

Vertebral Artery

Anterior Inferior Cerebellar Artery

Anterior Spinal Artery

Posterior Inferior Cerebellar Artery

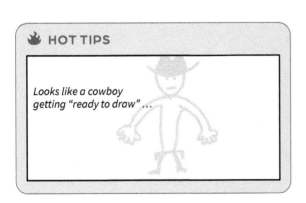

HOW TO ... DRAW VENOUS DRAINAGE OF THE HEAD

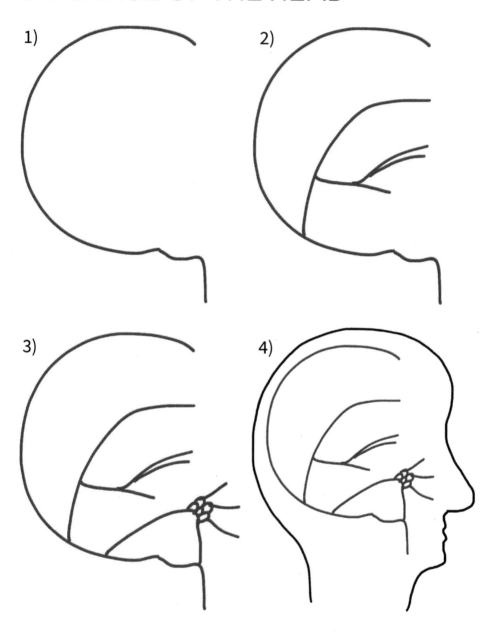

1)

2)

3)

4)

VENOUS DRAINAGE OF THE HEAD

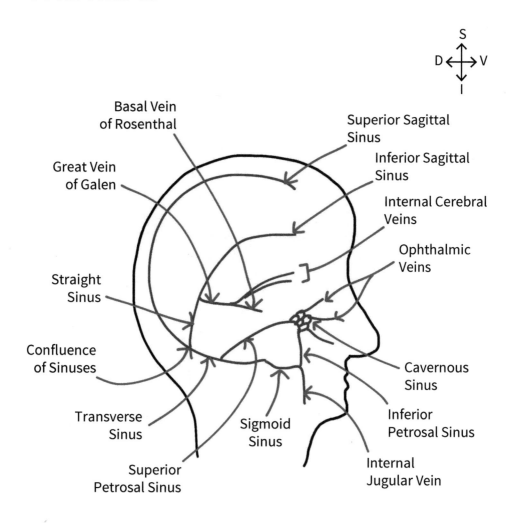

Basal Vein of Rosenthal

Great Vein of Galen

Straight Sinus

Confluence of Sinuses

Transverse Sinus

Superior Petrosal Sinus

Sigmoid Sinus

Superior Sagittal Sinus

Inferior Sagittal Sinus

Internal Cerebral Veins

Ophthalmic Veins

Cavernous Sinus

Inferior Petrosal Sinus

Internal Jugular Vein

S
D ← → V
I

> 🔥 **HOT TIPS**
> The sigmoid sinus becomes the internal jugular vein when it passes through the jugular foramen.

BLOOD SUPPLY TO BRAIN: LATERAL VIEW

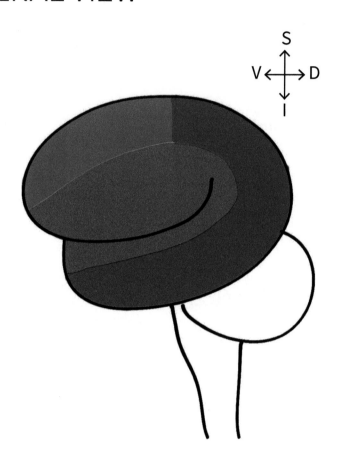

> 🔥 **HOT TIPS**
> Anterior Cerebral Artery: red.
> Middle Cerebral Artery: green.
> Posterior Cerebral Artery: blue.

BLOOD SUPPLY TO BRAIN: SAGITTAL VIEW

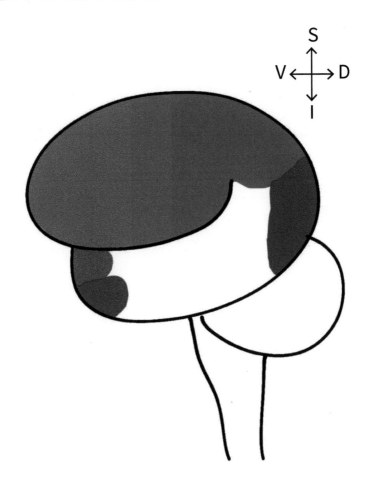

> 🔥 **HOT TIPS**
> Anterior Cerebral Artery: red.
> Middle Cerebral Artery: green.
> Posterior Cerebral Artery: blue.

HOW TO ... DRAW THE BRACHIAL PLEXUS

1)

2)

3)

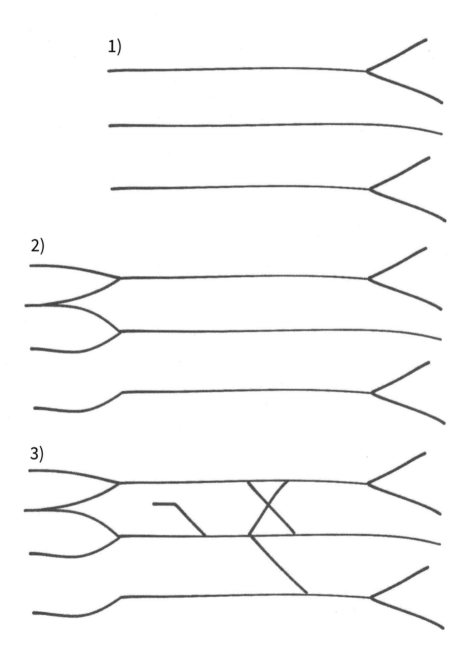

THE BRACHIAL PLEXUS

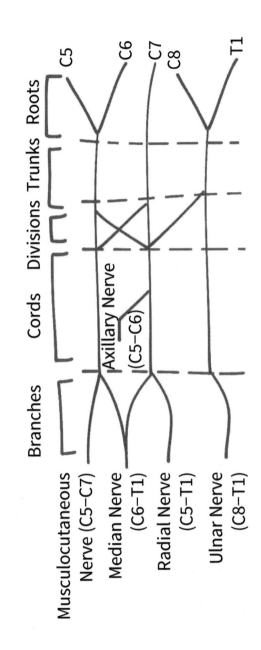

CHAPTER SEVEN

GENITOURINARY

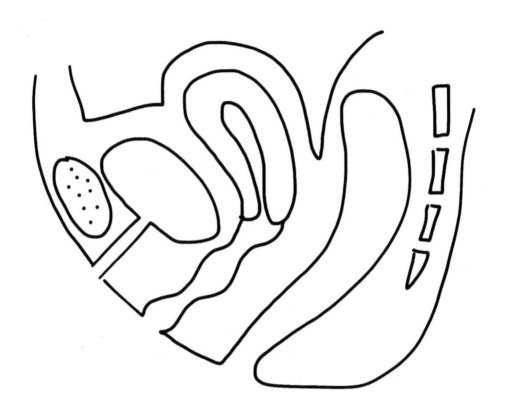

HOW TO ... DRAW THE KIDNEY

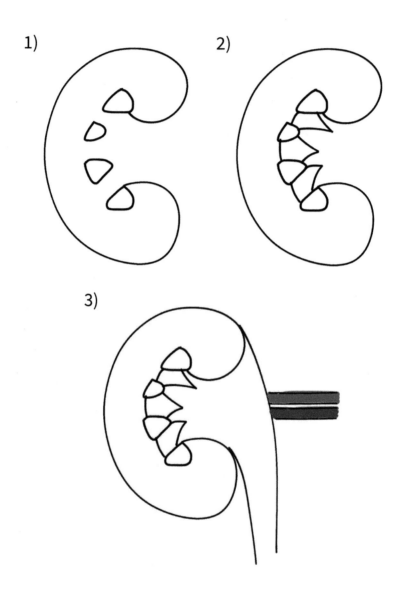

1)

2)

3)

ANATOMY OF THE KIDNEY

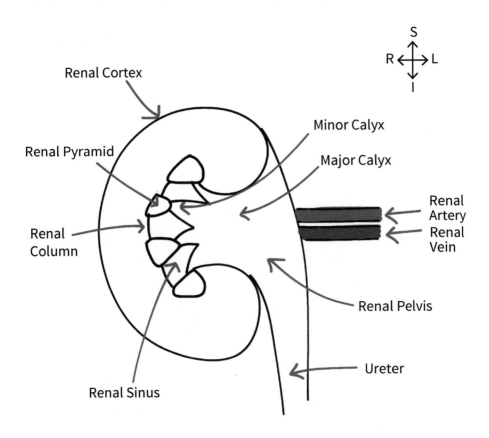

Renal Cortex

Renal Pyramid

Renal Column

Renal Sinus

Minor Calyx

Major Calyx

Renal Artery

Renal Vein

Renal Pelvis

Ureter

S
R ← → L
I

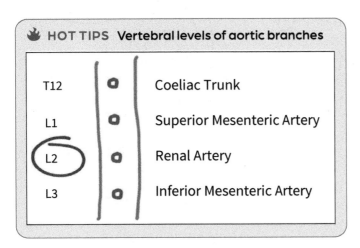

🔥 **HOT TIPS** **Vertebral levels of aortic branches**

T12	▢	Coeliac Trunk
L1	▢	Superior Mesenteric Artery
L2	▢	Renal Artery
L3	▢	Inferior Mesenteric Artery

HOW TO ... DRAW THE MALE REPRODUCTIVE SYSTEM

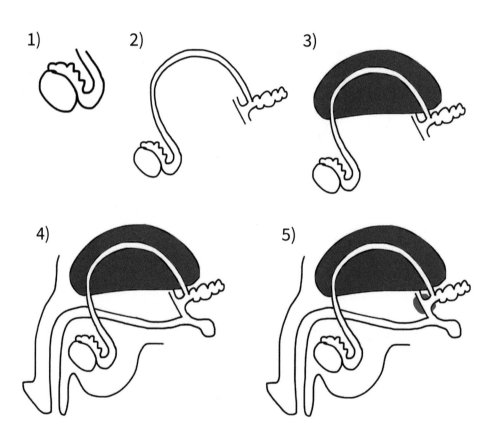

1)

2)

3)

4)

5)

THE MALE REPRODUCTIVE SYSTEM

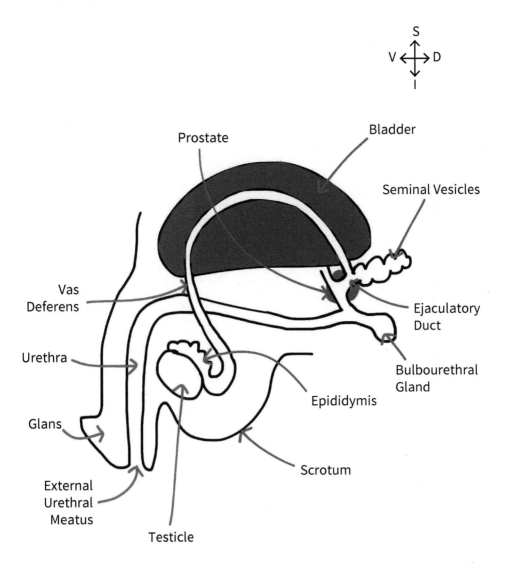

CROSS SECTION OF THE PENIS

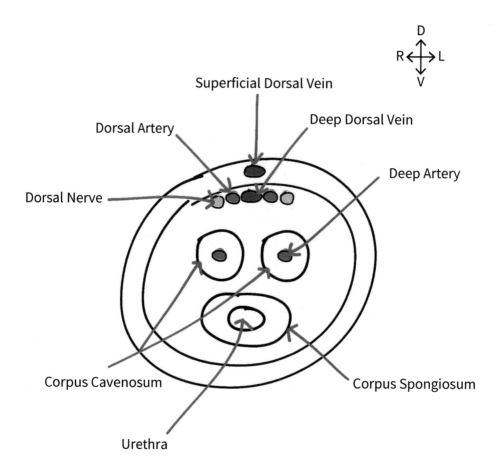

Superficial Dorsal Vein

Deep Dorsal Vein

Dorsal Artery

Deep Artery

Dorsal Nerve

Corpus Cavenosum

Corpus Spongiosum

Urethra

D
R ← → L
V

🔥 **HOT TIPS**

Layers of the Scrotum	(Remember)
Skin	Some
Dartos Muscle	Damn
External Spermatic Fascia	Englishman
Cremastic Fascia	Called
Internal Spermatic Fascia	It
Tunica Vaginalis	The
Tunica Albagenis	Testicle

HOW TO ... DRAW THE FEMALE REPRODUCTIVE SYSTEM

1)

2)

3)

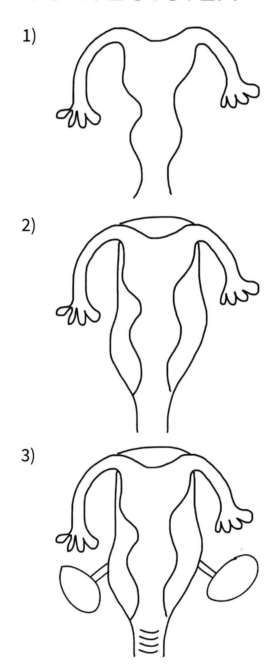

THE FEMALE REPRODUCTIVE SYSTEM

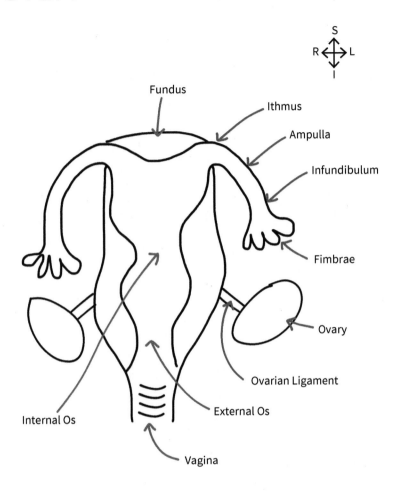

🔥 HOT TIPS

The Fallopian Tube is comprised of the:

- Isthmus
- Ampulla
- Infundibulum

The Broad Ligament (not shown here) is broad like its name suggests and looks like a cape.

HOW TO ... DRAW THE SURFACE ANATOMY OF FEMALE GENITALS

1)

2)

3)

4)

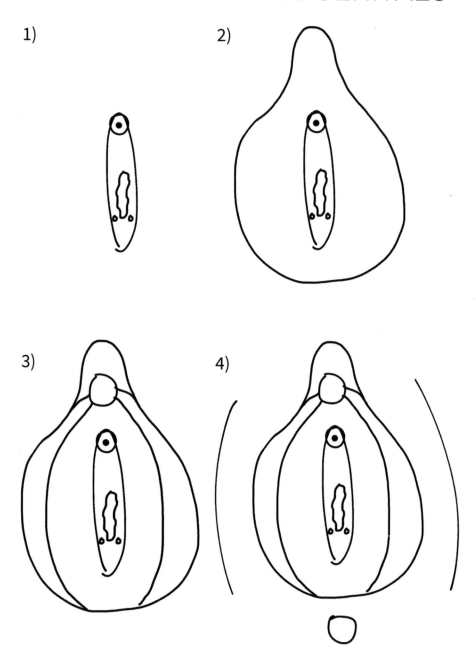

SURFACE ANATOMY OF FEMALE GENITALS

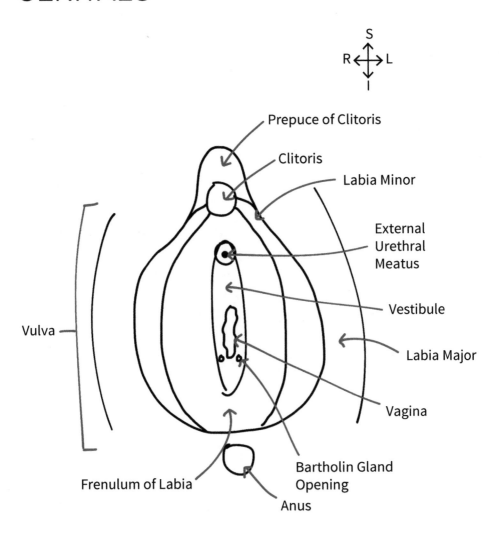

S

R ←→ L

I

Prepuce of Clitoris

Clitoris

Labia Minor

External
Urethral
Meatus

Vestibule

Labia Major

Vulva

Vagina

Frenulum of Labia

Bartholin Gland
Opening

Anus

HOW TO ... DRAW THE FEMALE PELVIC PERITONEUM

1)

2)

3)

4)

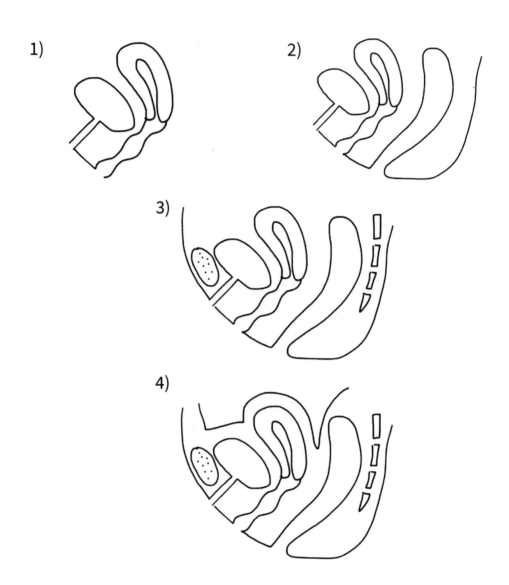

THE FEMALE PELVIC PERITONEUM

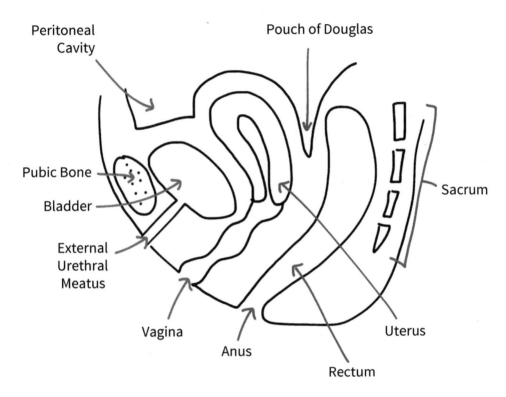

Peritoneal Cavity

Pouch of Douglas

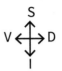

Pubic Bone

Bladder

External Urethral Meatus

Vagina

Anus

Rectum

Uterus

Sacrum

HOW TO ... DRAW THE BLADDER

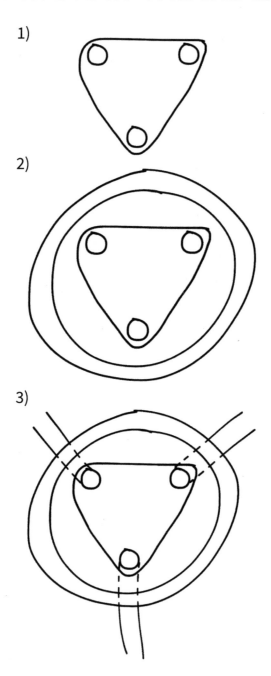

1)

2)

3)

THE BLADDER

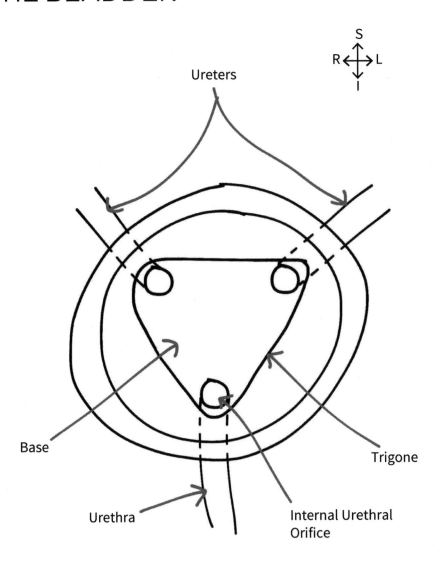

Ureters

S
R ← → L
I

Base

Urethra

Trigone

Internal Urethral Orifice

🔥 **HOT TIPS**

The Detrusor muscle is found in the wall of the bladder; it contracts to aid micturition (urination).

CHAPTER EIGHT

MUSCULOSKELETAL

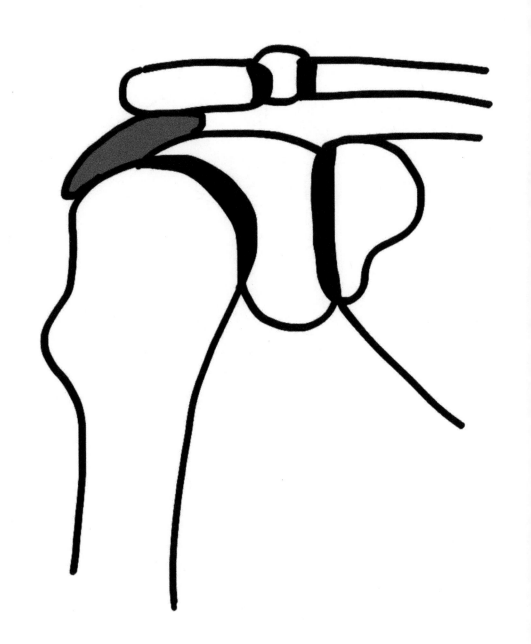

HOW TO ... DRAW THE FOOT

1)

2)

3)

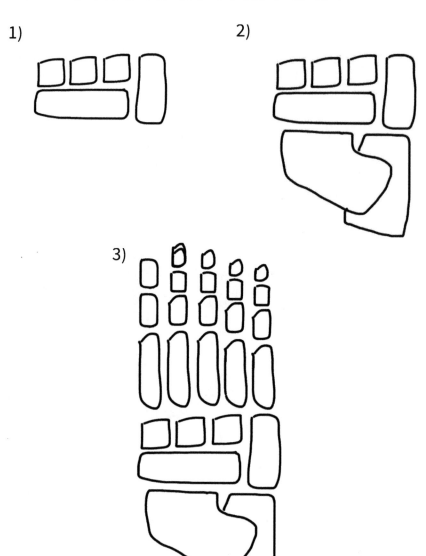

THE FOOT

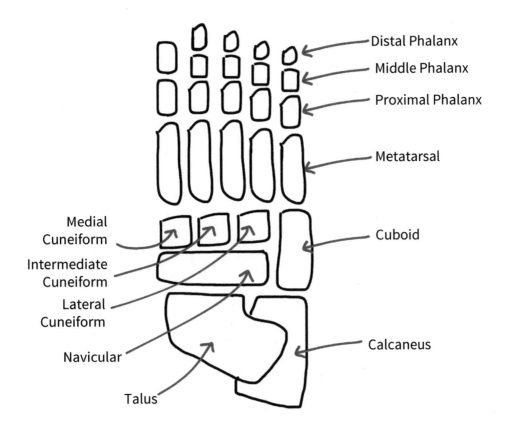

Distal Phalanx

Middle Phalanx

Proximal Phalanx

Metatarsal

Medial Cuneiform

Intermediate Cuneiform

Lateral Cuneiform

Navicular

Talus

Cuboid

Calcaneus

HOW TO ... DRAW THE HAND

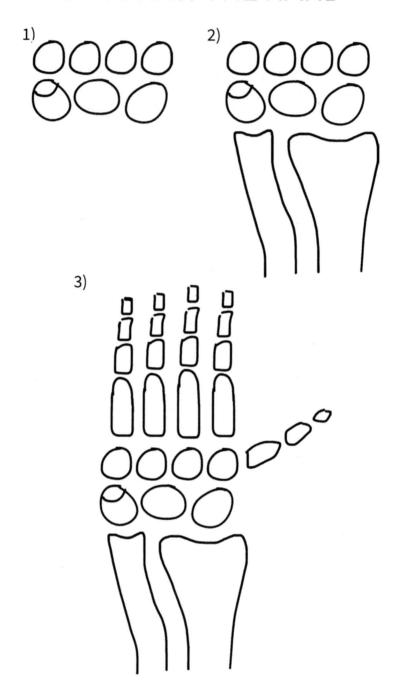

THE HAND

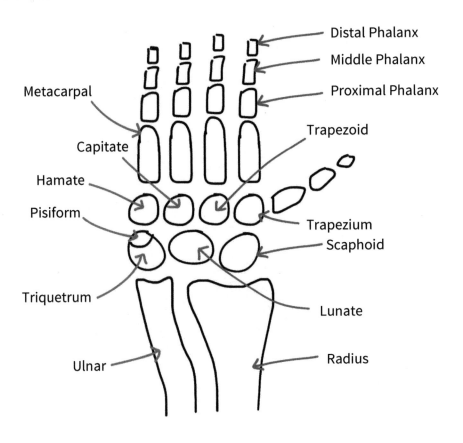

Distal Phalanx

Middle Phalanx

Proximal Phalanx

Metacarpal

Trapezoid

Capitate

Hamate

Pisiform

Trapezium

Scaphoid

Triquetrum

Lunate

Ulnar

Radius

🔥 **HOT TIPS**

How to remember the bones in the hand

'So Long To Pinky, Here Comes The Thumb'

'Scaphoid, Lunate, Triquetrum, Hamate, Capitate, Trapezoid, and Trapezium'

'The TrapeziUM joins the ThUMb.'

HOW TO ... DRAW THE CARPAL TUNNEL

1)

2)

3)

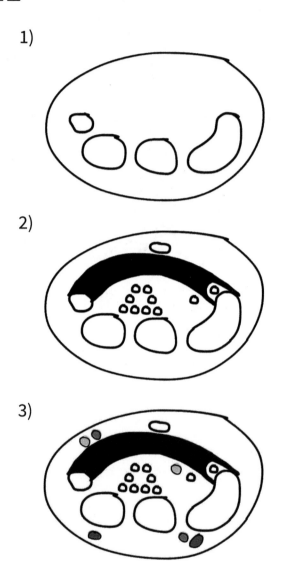

THE CARPAL TUNNEL

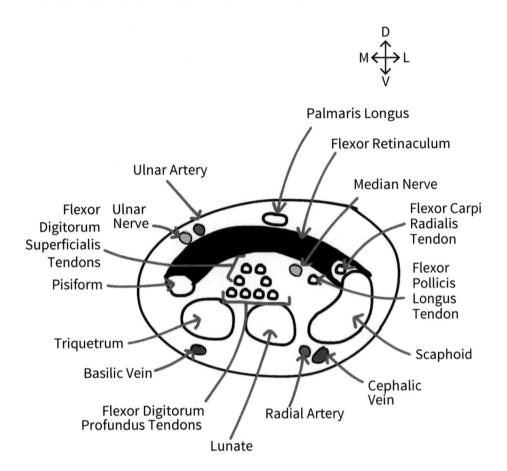

D
M ← → L
V

Palmaris Longus

Flexor Retinaculum

Ulnar Artery

Median Nerve

Flexor Digitorum Superficialis Tendons

Ulnar Nerve

Flexor Carpi Radialis Tendon

Pisiform

Flexor Pollicis Longus Tendon

Triquetrum

Basilic Vein

Scaphoid

Flexor Digitorum Profundus Tendons

Cephalic Vein

Radial Artery

Lunate

HOW TO ... DRAW THE KNEE

1)

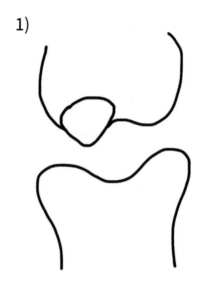

2)

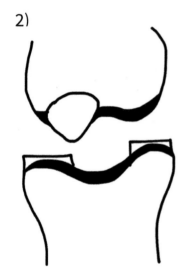

3)

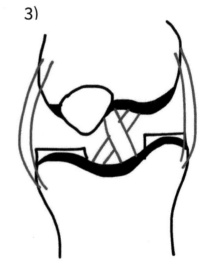

KNEE ANATOMY

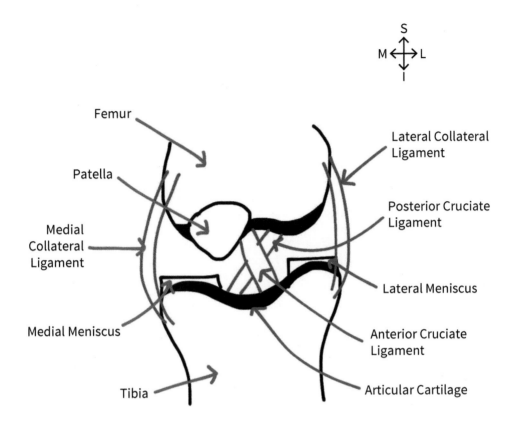

S
M ←→ L
I

Femur

Patella

Medial Collateral Ligament

Medial Meniscus

Tibia

Lateral Collateral Ligament

Posterior Cruciate Ligament

Lateral Meniscus

Anterior Cruciate Ligament

Articular Cartilage

HOW TO ... DRAW THE HIP

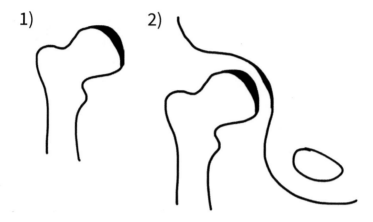

1)

2)

THE HIP

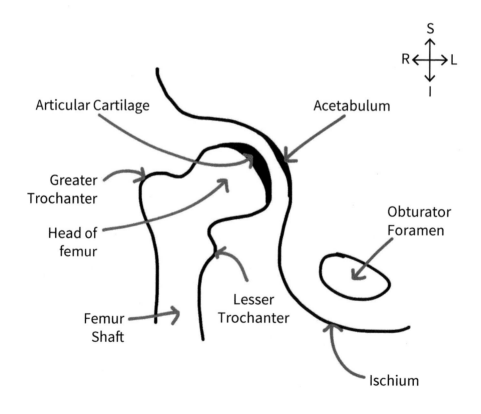

Articular Cartilage

Acetabulum

Greater Trochanter

Head of femur

Obturator Foramen

Femur Shaft

Lesser Trochanter

Ischium

S
R ← → L
I

HIP AND FEMUR ANATOMY

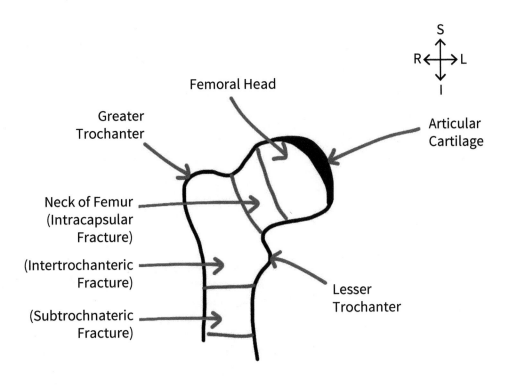

Femoral Head

Greater Trochanter

Articular Cartilage

Neck of Femur (Intracapsular Fracture)

(Intertrochanteric Fracture)

(Subtrochnateric Fracture)

Lesser Trochanter

S

R ← → L

I

🔥 **HOT TIPS**

Intertrochanteric and Subtrochanteric fractures are both extracapsular fractures, i.e. they do not include the femoral head or neck.

HOW TO ... DRAW THE SHOULDER

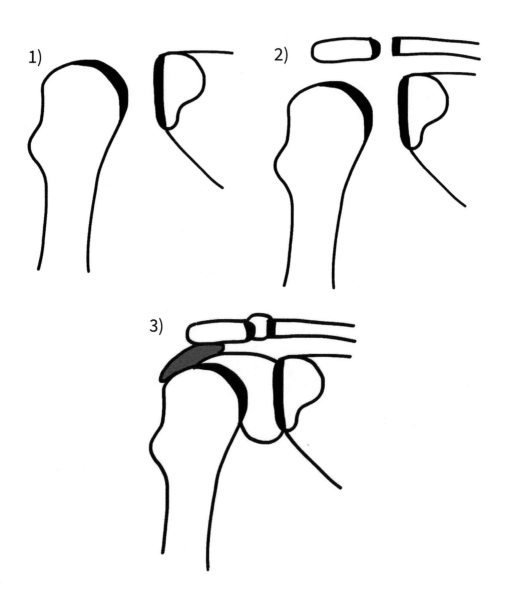

1)

2)

3)

THE SHOULDER

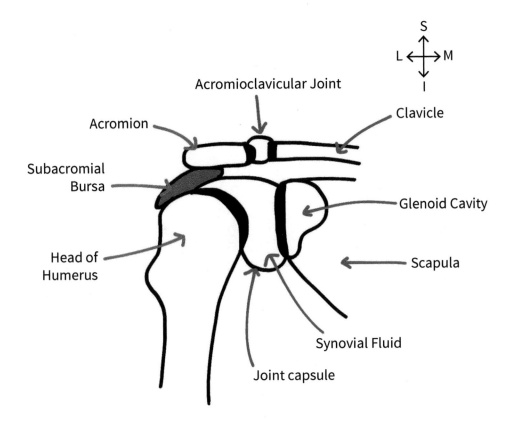

S
L ←→ M
I

Acromioclavicular Joint

Acromion

Clavicle

Subacromial
Bursa

Glenoid Cavity

Head of
Humerus

Scapula

Synovial Fluid

Joint capsule

🔥 HOT TIPS

Remember: the acromion is a part of the scapula—unlike demonstrated here where it looks like it is not.

HOW TO ... DRAW THE ELBOW

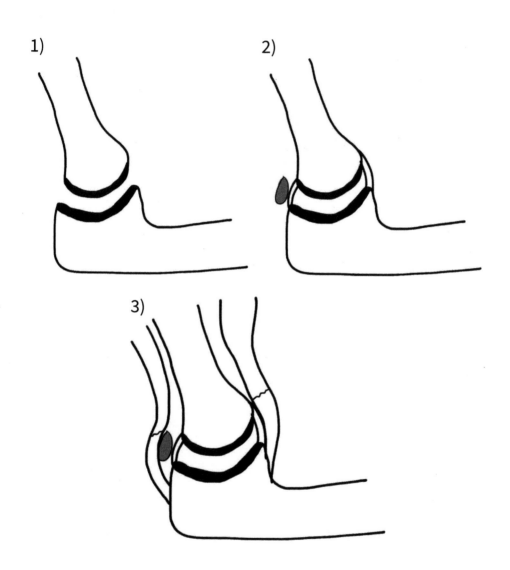

1)

2)

3)

THE ELBOW

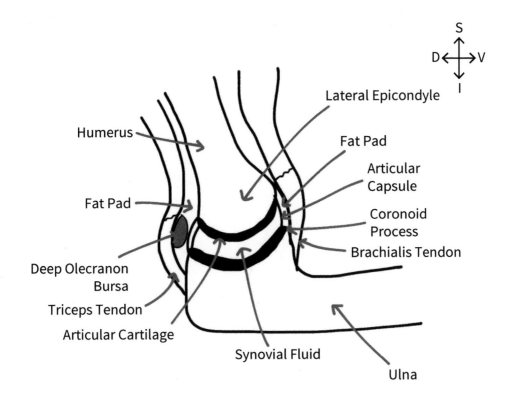

Lateral Epicondyle

Humerus

Fat Pad

Articular Capsule

Fat Pad

Coronoid Process

Brachialis Tendon

Deep Olecranon Bursa

Triceps Tendon

Articular Cartilage

Synovial Fluid

Ulna

S
D ← → V
I

🔥 **HOT TIPS**
The Radius is not shown in this diagram but forms part of the elbow.

HOW TO ... DRAW THE SCAPULA

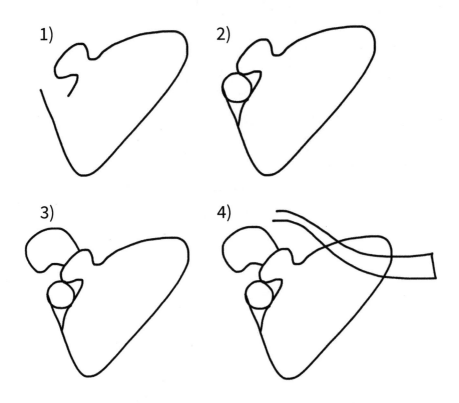

1)

2)

3)

4)

THE SCAPULA

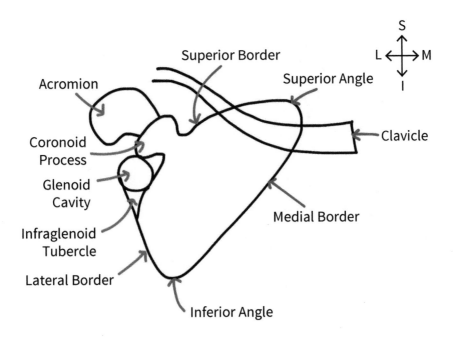

HOW TO ... DRAW LIGAMENTS OF THE SHOULDER

1)

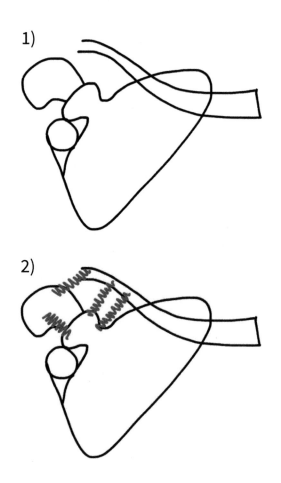

2)

THE SHOULDER LIGAMENTS

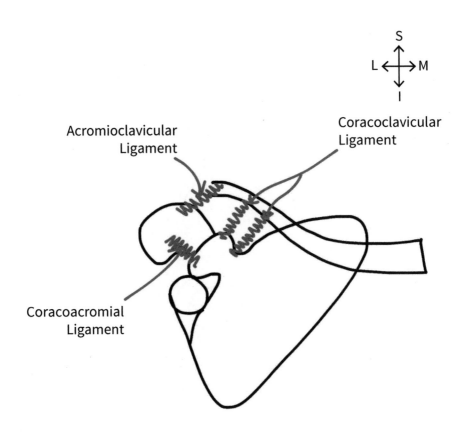

Acromioclavicular Ligament

Coracoclavicular Ligament

Coracoacromial Ligament

S
L ← → M
I

HOW TO ... DRAW MUSCLES OF THE SCAPULA (POSTERIOR VIEW)

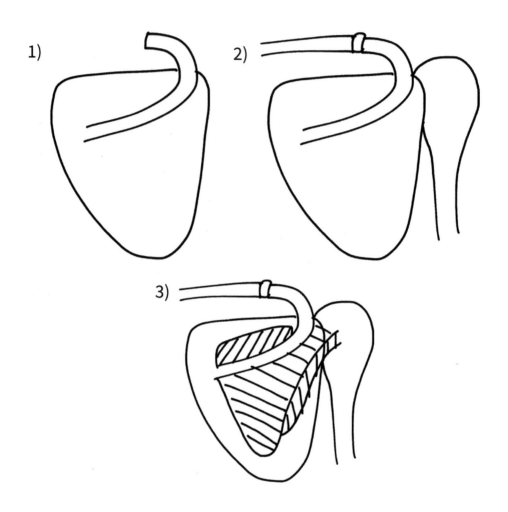

1)

2)

3)

MUSCLES OF THE SCAPULA: POSTERIOR VIEW

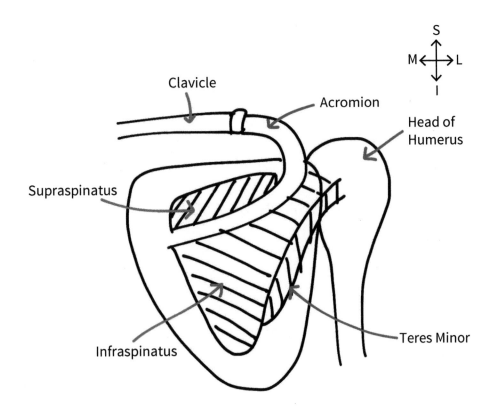

S

M ← → L

I

Clavicle

Acromion

Head of Humerus

Supraspinatus

Teres Minor

Infraspinatus

🔥 **HOT TIPS**

The Subscapularis muscle lies on the other side of the Scapula not shown in this view.

SPINE ANATOMY: LATERAL VIEW

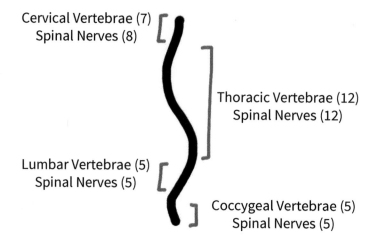

Cervical Vertebrae (7)
Spinal Nerves (8)

Thoracic Vertebrae (12)
Spinal Nerves (12)

Lumbar Vertebrae (5)
Spinal Nerves (5)

Coccygeal Vertebrae (5)
Spinal Nerves (5)

VERTEBRA ANATOMY: SUPERIOR VIEW

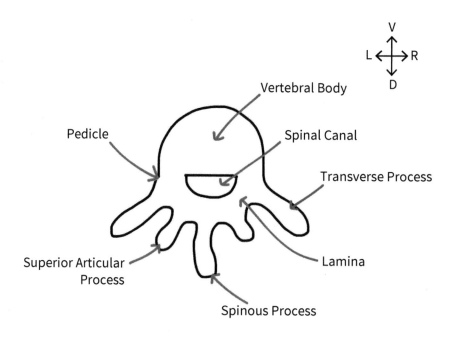

Vertebral Body

Pedicle

Spinal Canal

Transverse Process

Superior Articular
Process

Lamina

Spinous Process

CHAPTER NINE
OPHTHALMOLOGY

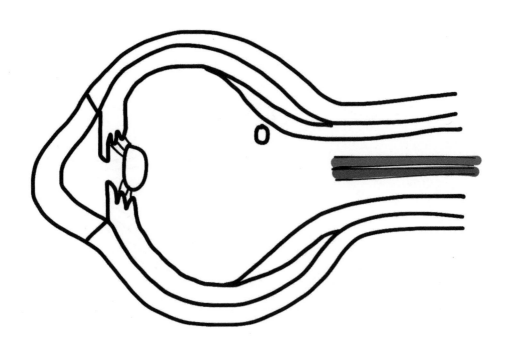

HOW TO … DRAW CROSS SECTION OF THE EYE

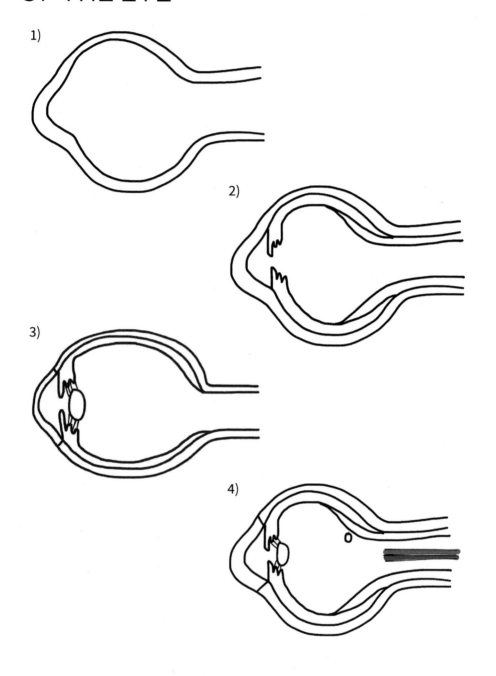

1)

2)

3)

4)

CROSS SECTION OF THE EYE

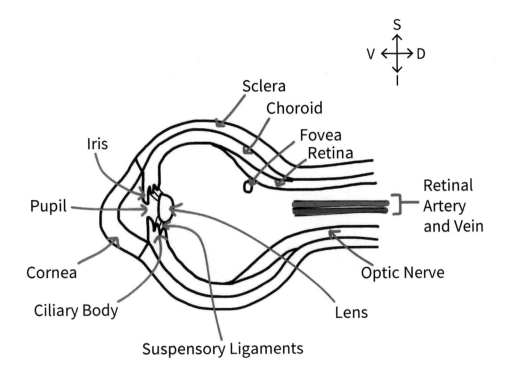

EYE MUSCLES AND MOVEMENT

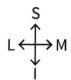

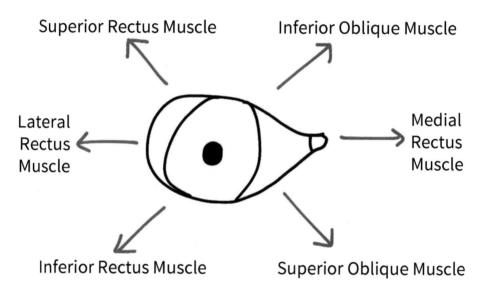

Superior Rectus Muscle

Inferior Oblique Muscle

Lateral Rectus Muscle

Medial Rectus Muscle

Inferior Rectus Muscle

Superior Oblique Muscle

🔥 **HOT TIPS**

How to remember eye movements and cranial nerves

Think SO4 LR6:

   Superior oblique innervated by cranial nerve 4 (trochlear).

   Lateral rectus innervated by cranial nerve 6 (abducens).

CHAPTER TEN

MISCELLANEOUS

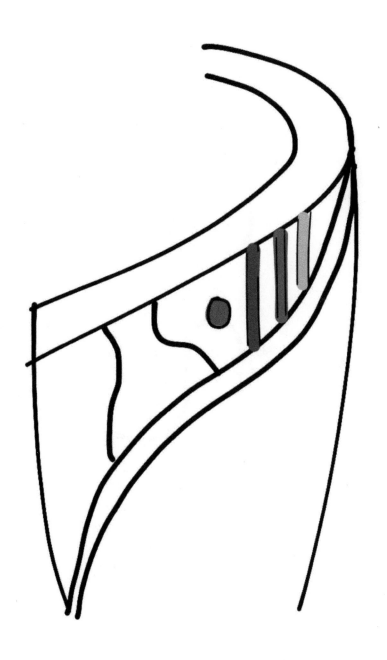

HOW TO … DRAW THE THYROID GLAND

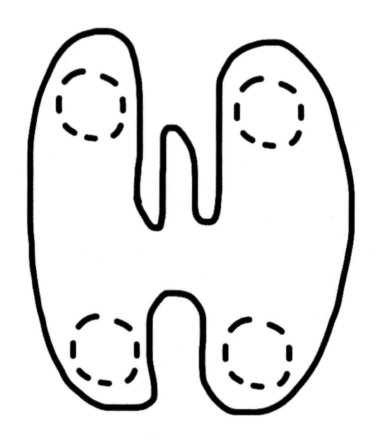

THE THYROID GLAND

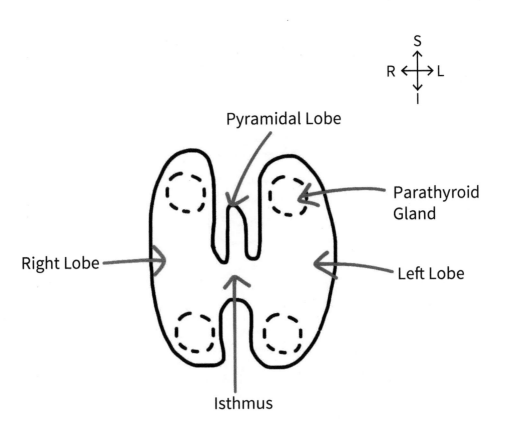

S

R ←→ L

I

Pyramidal Lobe

Parathyroid Gland

Right Lobe

Left Lobe

Isthmus

HOW TO ... DRAW TRANSVERSE SECTION OF THE ANTERIOR NECK

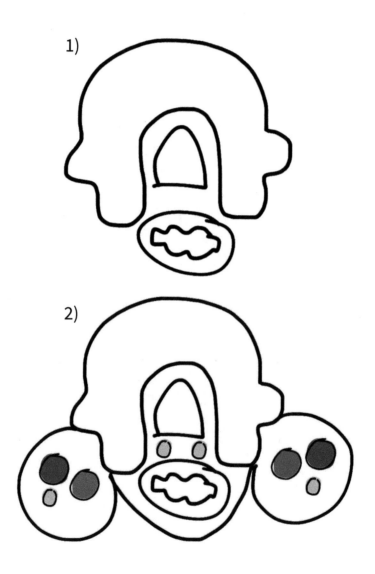

1)

2)

TRANSVERSE SECTION OF THE ANTERIOR NECK

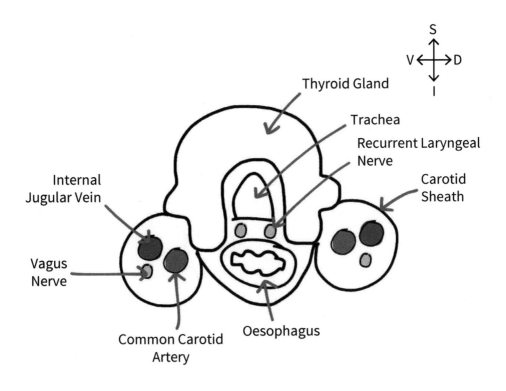

S
V ← → D
I

Thyroid Gland

Trachea

Recurrent Laryngeal Nerve

Carotid Sheath

Internal Jugular Vein

Vagus Nerve

Common Carotid Artery

Oesophagus

🔥 **HOT TIPS** **Carotid sheath**

Contains the
- Common Carotid Artery, Internal Jugular Vein and Vagus Nerve.

HOW TO … DRAW THE FEMORAL TRIANGLE

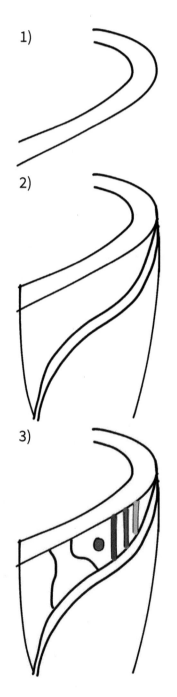

1)

2)

3)

THE FEMORAL TRIANGLE

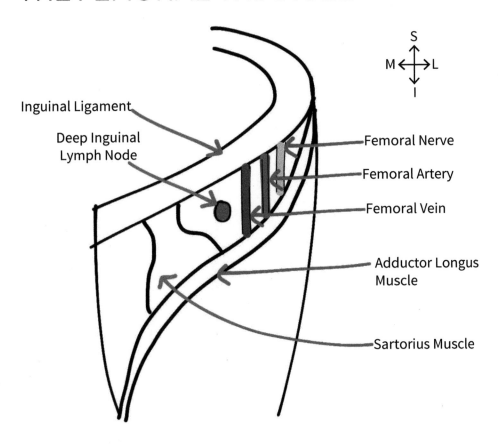

Inguinal Ligament

Deep Inguinal
Lymph Node

Femoral Nerve

Femoral Artery

Femoral Vein

Adductor Longus
Muscle

Sartorius Muscle

S

M ← → L

I

🔥 **HOT TIPS** **Femoral triangle borders**
Superior border: the Inguinal Ligament.
Lateral border: medial border of the Sartorius Muscle.
Medial border: medial border of the Adductor Longus Muscle.
Think NAVY:

Nerve

Artery

Vein

LYmph node.

HOW TO ... DRAW THE ANTERIOR CUBITAL FOSSA

1)

2)

3)

4)

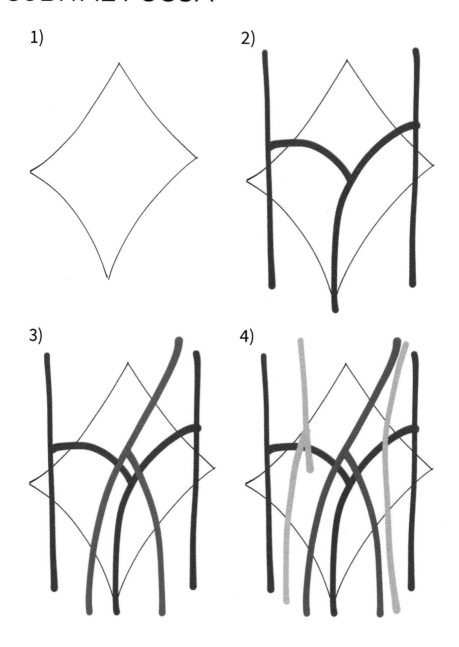

THE ANTERIOR CUBITAL FOSSA

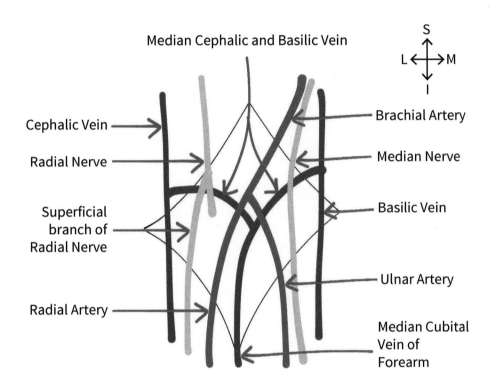

Median Cephalic and Basilic Vein

S
L ← → M
I

Cephalic Vein

Radial Nerve

Superficial branch of Radial Nerve

Radial Artery

Brachial Artery

Median Nerve

Basilic Vein

Ulnar Artery

Median Cubital Vein of Forearm

🔥 **HOT TIPS** **Median cubital vein**
The Median Cubital Vein is usually used for phlebotomy (collection of blood) and is located in the anterior aspect of the elbow.

HOW TO ... DRAW ARTERY SUPPLY OF THE (RIGHT) LEG

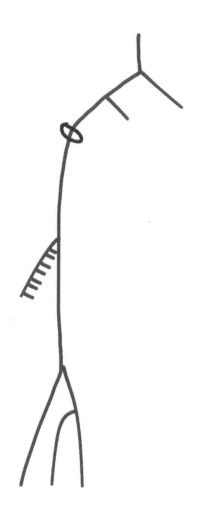

ARTERY SUPPLY OF THE (RIGHT) LEG

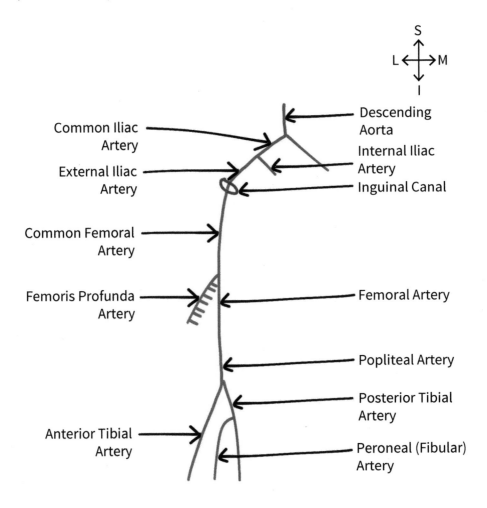

S

L ← → M

I

Common Iliac Artery

External Iliac Artery

Common Femoral Artery

Femoris Profunda Artery

Anterior Tibial Artery

Descending Aorta

Internal Iliac Artery

Inguinal Canal

Femoral Artery

Popliteal Artery

Posterior Tibial Artery

Peroneal (Fibular) Artery

HOW TO ... DRAW VENOUS DRAINAGE OF THE (LEFT) LEG

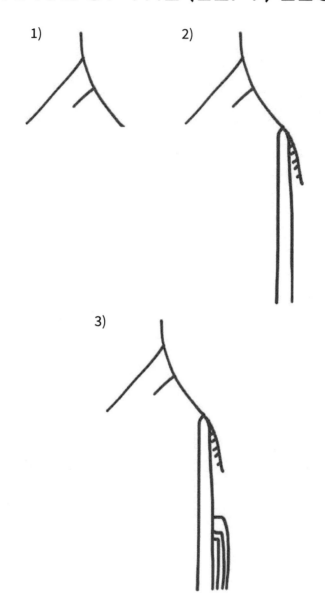

1)

2)

3)

VENOUS DRAINAGE OF THE (LEFT) LEG

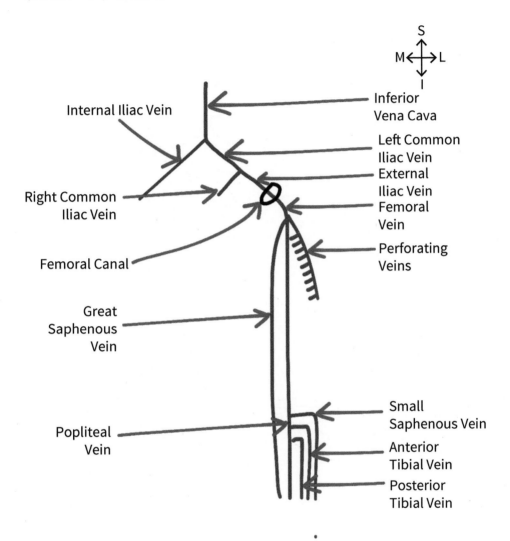

HOW TO ... DRAW THE BREAST

1)

2)

3)

4)

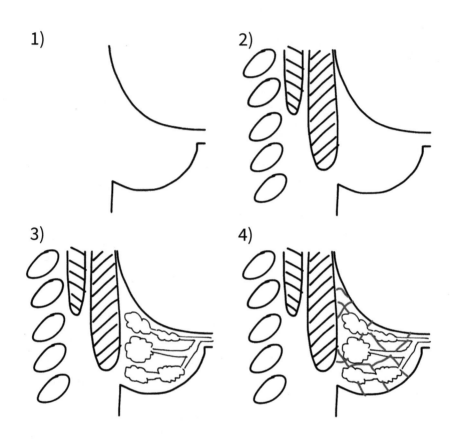

THE BREAST

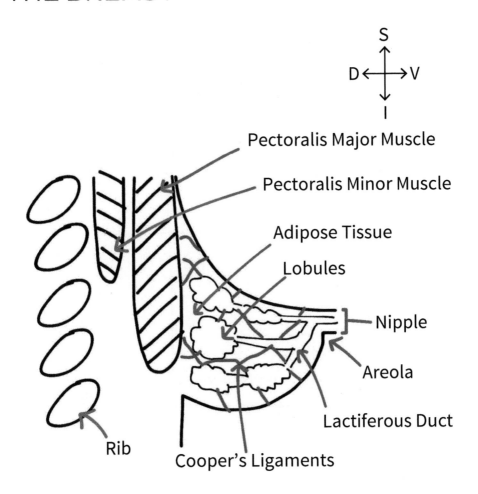

S

D ← → V

I

Pectoralis Major Muscle

Pectoralis Minor Muscle

Adipose Tissue

Lobules

Nipple

Areola

Lactiferous Duct

Rib

Cooper's Ligaments

HOW TO ... DRAW AREAS OF ABDOMEN

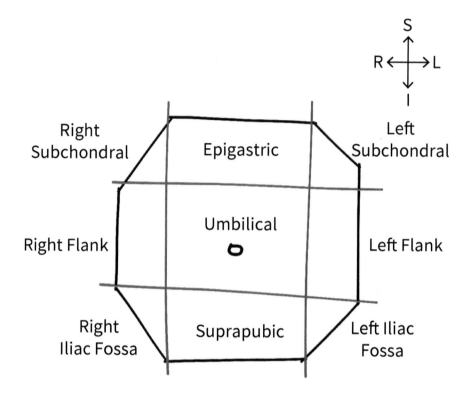

HOW TO ... DRAW SURGICAL SCARS

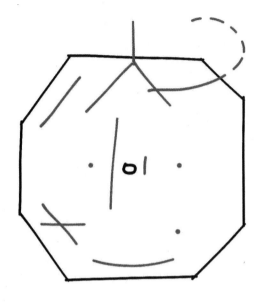

SURGICAL SCARS

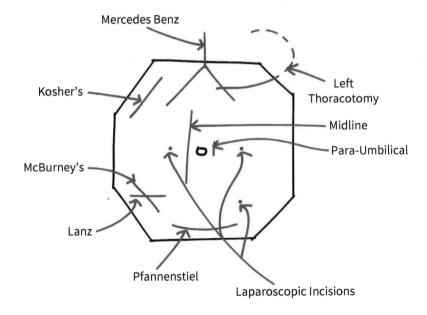

Mercedes Benz

Kosher's

Left
Thoracotomy

Midline

Para-Umbilical

McBurney's

Lanz

Pfannenstiel

Laparoscopic Incisions

CHAPTER ELEVEN

RESPIRATORY HISTOLOGY

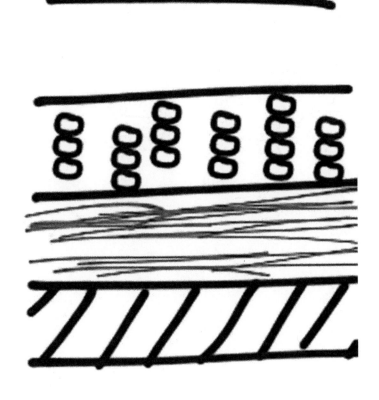

HOW TO ... DRAW THE TRACHEA HISTOLOGY

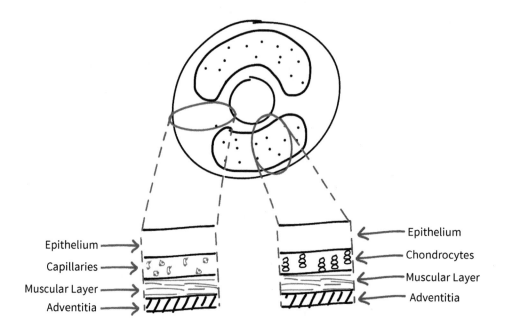

Epithelium
Capillaries
Muscular Layer
Adventitia

Epithelium
Chondrocytes
Muscular Layer
Adventitia

 HOT TIPS
Tracheal Epithelium is columnar, pseudostratified and ciliated.

CHAPTER TWELVE

GASTROINTESTINAL TRACT HISTOLOGY

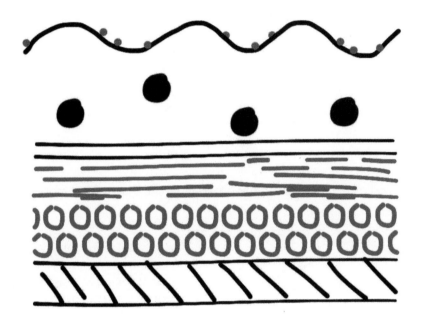

HOW TO ... DRAW THE GASTROINTESTINAL TRACT HISTOLOGY

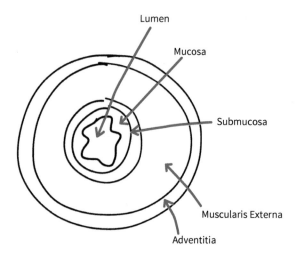

Lumen

Mucosa

Submucosa

Muscularis Externa

Adventitia

(When we flatten the tube out this allows us to see the layers in more detail.)

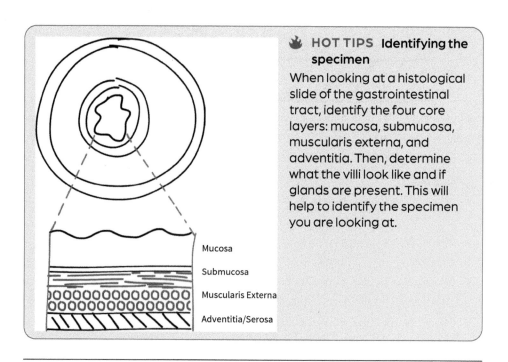

Mucosa

Submucosa

Muscularis Externa

Adventitia/Serosa

🔥 **HOT TIPS** **Identifying the specimen**

When looking at a histological slide of the gastrointestinal tract, identify the four core layers: mucosa, submucosa, muscularis externa, and adventitia. Then, determine what the villi look like and if glands are present. This will help to identify the specimen you are looking at.

HOW TO ... DRAW THE STOMACH HISTOLOGY

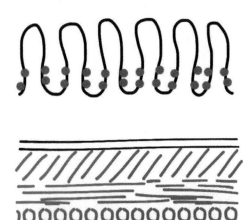

THE STOMACH HISTOLOGY

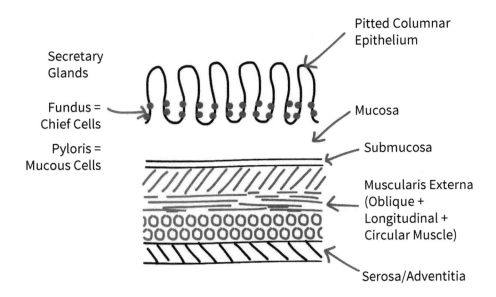

Secretary Glands

Fundus = Chief Cells

Pyloris = Mucous Cells

Pitted Columnar Epithelium

Mucosa

Submucosa

Muscularis Externa (Oblique + Longitudinal + Circular Muscle)

Serosa/Adventitia

HOW TO ... DRAW THE DUODENUM HISTOLOGY

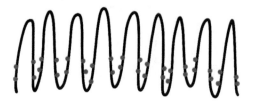

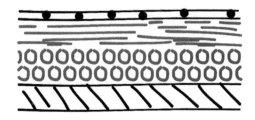

THE DUODENUM HISTOLOGY

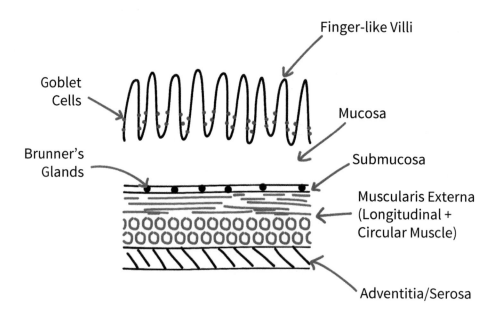

Finger-like Villi

Goblet
Cells

Mucosa

Brunner's
Glands

Submucosa

Muscularis Externa
(Longitudinal +
Circular Muscle)

Adventitia/Serosa

HOW TO ... DRAW THE JEJUNUM HISTOLOGY

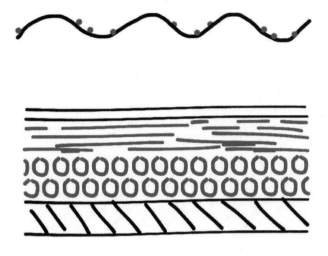

THE JEJUNUM HISTOLOGY

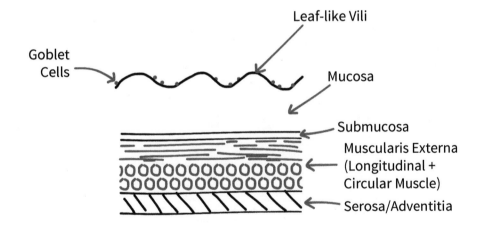

Leaf-like Vili

Goblet Cells

Mucosa

Submucosa

Muscularis Externa (Longitudinal + Circular Muscle)

Serosa/Adventitia

HOW TO ... DRAW THE ILEUM HISTOLOGY

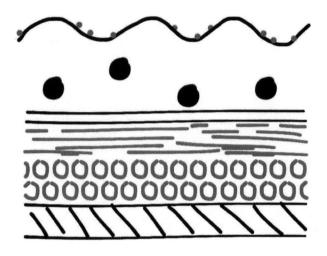

THE ILEUM HISTOLOGY

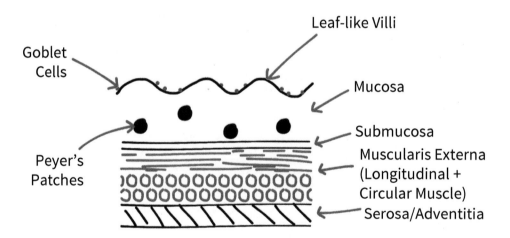

Leaf-like Villi

Goblet Cells

Mucosa

Submucosa

Peyer's Patches

Muscularis Externa (Longitudinal + Circular Muscle)

Serosa/Adventitia

HOW TO ... DRAW THE COLON HISTOLOGY

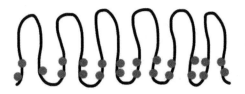

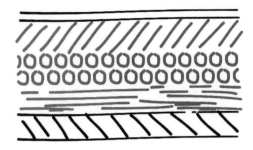

THE COLON HISTOLOGY

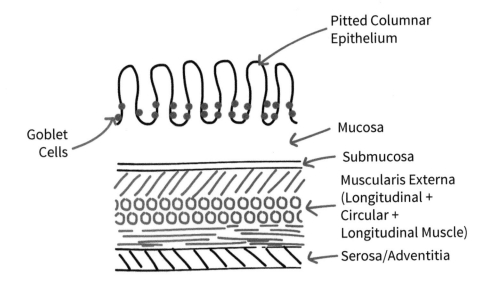

Pitted Columnar Epithelium

Goblet Cells

Mucosa

Submucosa

Muscularis Externa (Longitudinal + Circular + Longitudinal Muscle)

Serosa/Adventitia

CHAPTER THIRTEEN
HEPATIC
HISTOLOGY

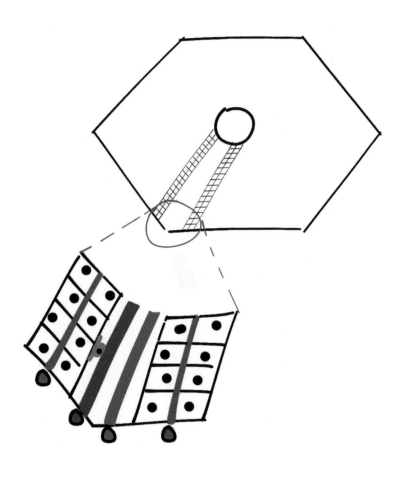

HOW TO ... DRAW LIVER HISTOLOGY

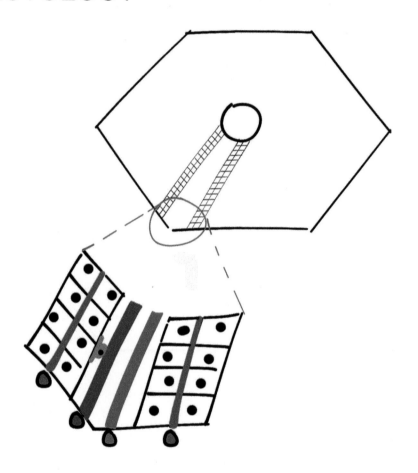

LIVER HISTOLOGY

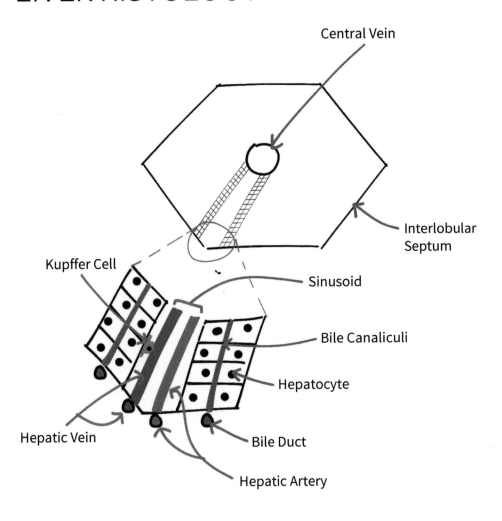

Central Vein

Interlobular Septum

Kupffer Cell

Sinusoid

Bile Canaliculi

Hepatocyte

Hepatic Vein

Bile Duct

Hepatic Artery

🔥 **HOT TIPS**

Liver is made by millions of these hexagonal lobules.

Remember: in this diagram bile flows downwards (out of the liver) and blood flows upwards (into the liver).

CHAPTER FOURTEEN
RENAL HISTOLOGY

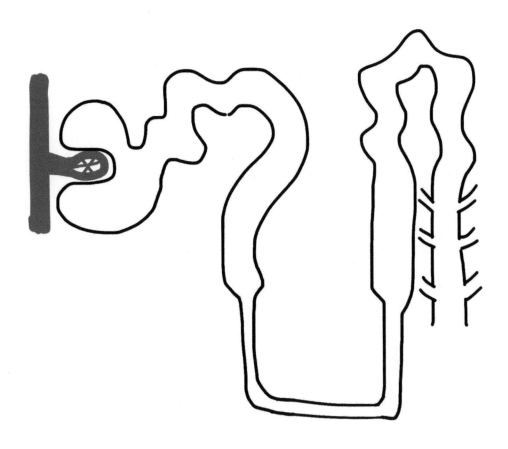

HOW TO ... DRAW THE LOOP OF HENLE

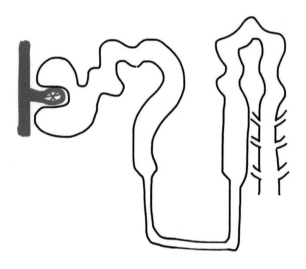

THE LOOP OF HENLE

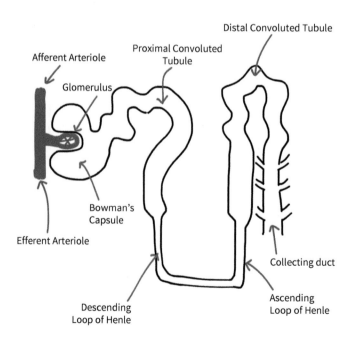

HOW TO ... DRAW THE ADRENAL GLAND HISTOLOGY

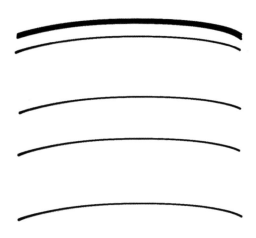

THE ADRENAL GLAND HISTOLOGY

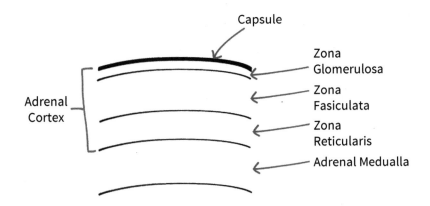

Capsule

Zona Glomerulosa

Zona Fasiculata

Adrenal Cortex

Zona Reticularis

Adrenal Medualla

 HOT TIPS

Remember: 'The deeper it goes, the sweeter it gets'.

- Mineralocorticoids (Glomerulosa)—salt.
- Glucocorticoids (Fasciulata)—sugar.
- Androgens (Reticularis)—sex hormones.

Think 'GFR' to remember the order of cortex.

CHAPTER FIFTEEN

MUSCULOSKELETAL HISTOLOGY

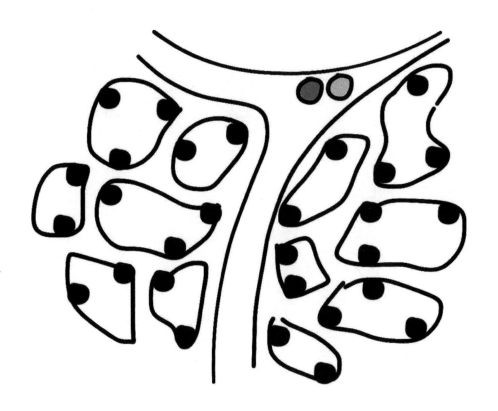

HOW TO ... DRAW MUSCLE FILAMENT LAYERS

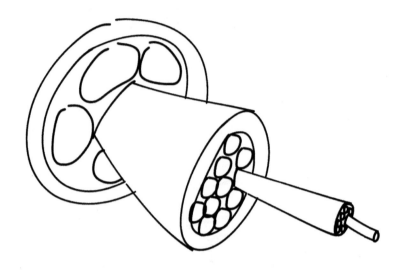

MUSCLE FILAMENT LAYERS

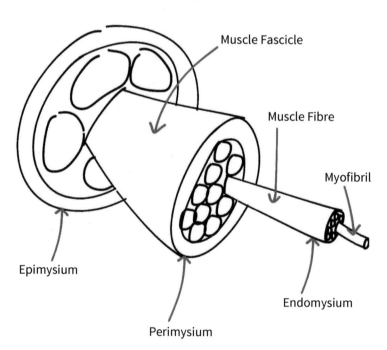

Muscle Fascicle

Muscle Fibre

Myofibril

Epimysium

Endomysium

Perimysium

HOW TO ... DRAW SKELETAL MUSCLE HISTOLOGY

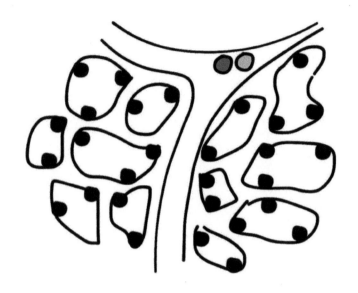

SKELETAL MUSCLE HISTOLOGY

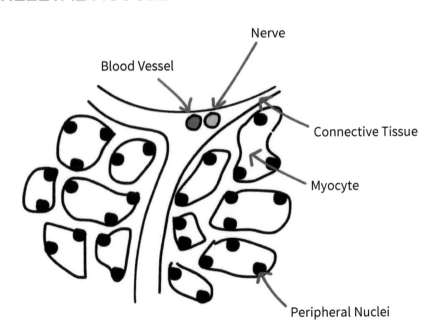

CHAPTER SIXTEEN

SKIN HISTOLOGY

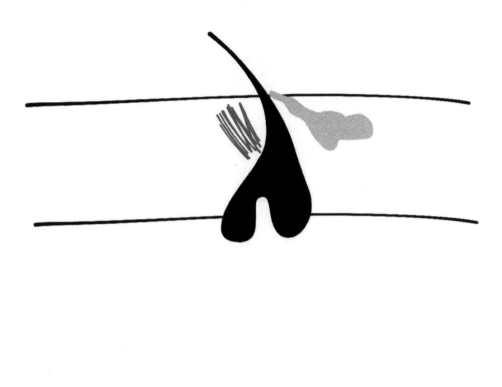

HOW TO ... DRAW THE HAIR FOLLICLE HISTOLOGY

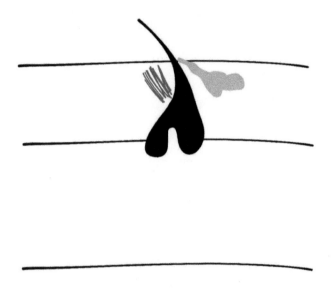

THE HAIR FOLLICLE HISTOLOGY

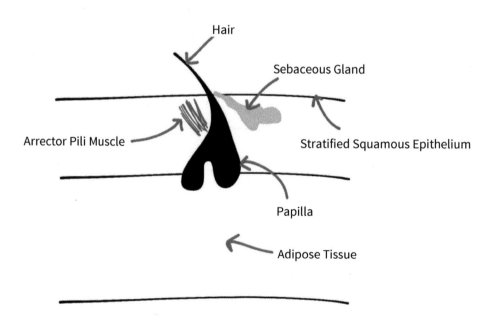

Hair

Sebaceous Gland

Arrector Pili Muscle

Stratified Squamous Epithelium

Papilla

Adipose Tissue

HOW TO … DRAW THICK SKIN HISTOLOGY

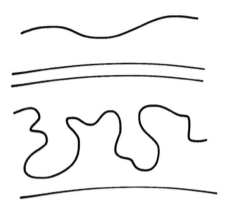

THICK SKIN HISTOLOGY

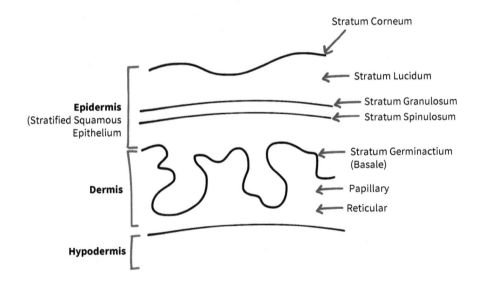

Stratum Corneum

Stratum Lucidum

Stratum Granulosum

Stratum Spinulosum

Epidermis
(Stratified Squamous
Epithelium

Stratum Germinactium
(Basale)

Dermis

Papillary

Reticular

Hypodermis

🔥 **HOT TIPS**

Thick skin (found on palms and soles of feet) contains Stratum Lucidium, whereas skin found elsewhere on the body lacks this layer.

HOW TO ... DRAW PACINIAN CORPUSCLES

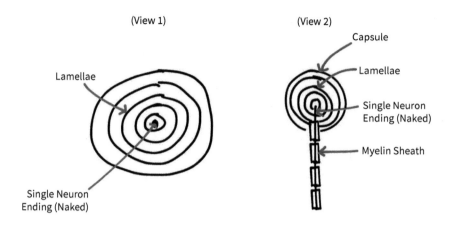

(View 1)

Lamellae

Single Neuron
Ending (Naked)

(View 2)

Capsule

Lamellae

Single Neuron
Ending (Naked)

Myelin Sheath

HOW TO ... DRAW MEISSNER'S CORPUSCLES

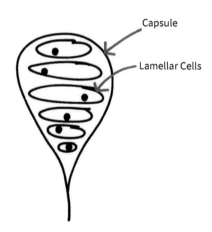

Capsule

Lamellar Cells

🔥 **HOT TIPS**

Depending on the section given, they may look like view 1 or view 2.

Function of Pacinian Corpuscles: detect **pressure**.

Function of Meissner's Corpuscles: detect **touch**.

CHAPTER SEVENTEEN

OPHTHALMIC HISTOLOGY

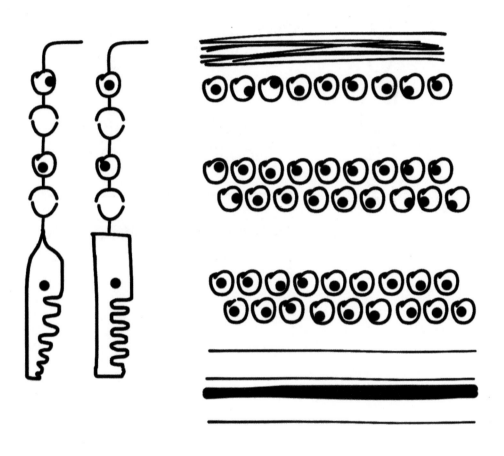

HOW TO … DRAW RETINAL HISTOLOGY

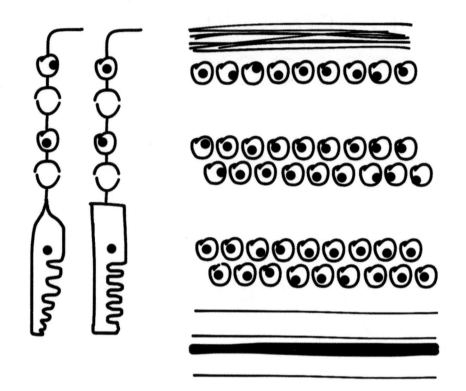

HISTOLOGY OF THE RETINA

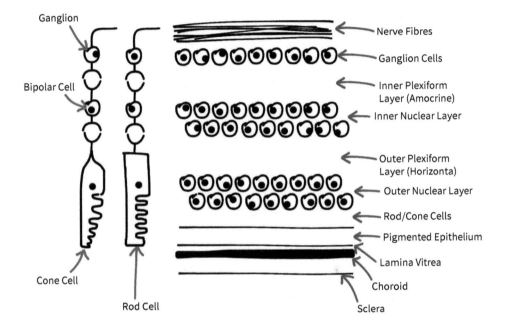

Ganglion

Bipolar Cell

Cone Cell

Rod Cell

Nerve Fibres

Ganglion Cells

Inner Plexiform
Layer (Amocrine)

Inner Nuclear Layer

Outer Plexiform
Layer (Horizonta)

Outer Nuclear Layer

Rod/Cone Cells

Pigmented Epithelium

Lamina Vitrea

Choroid

Sclera

CHAPTER EIGHTEEN

MISCELLANEOUS HISTOLOGY

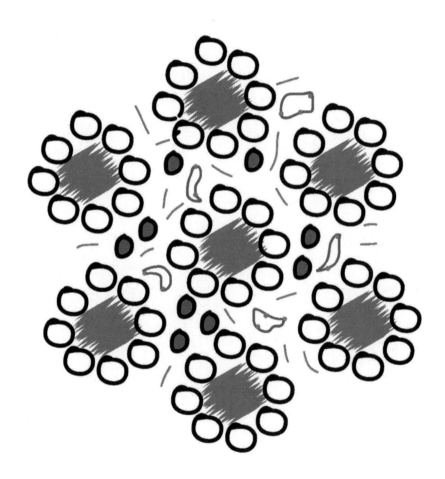

HOW TO ... DRAW THE THYROID GLAND HISTOLOGY

1)

2)

3)

4)

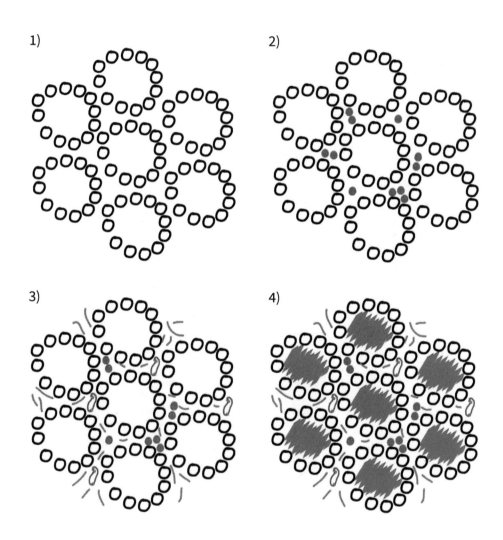

THE THYROID GLAND HISTOLOGY

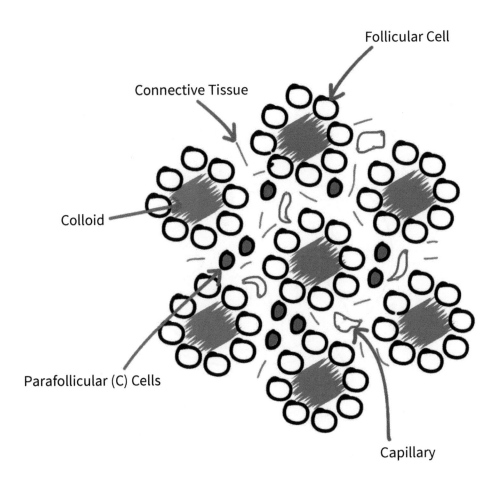

Follicular Cell

Connective Tissue

Colloid

Parafollicular (C) Cells

Capillary

HOW TO ... DRAW A LYMPH NODE

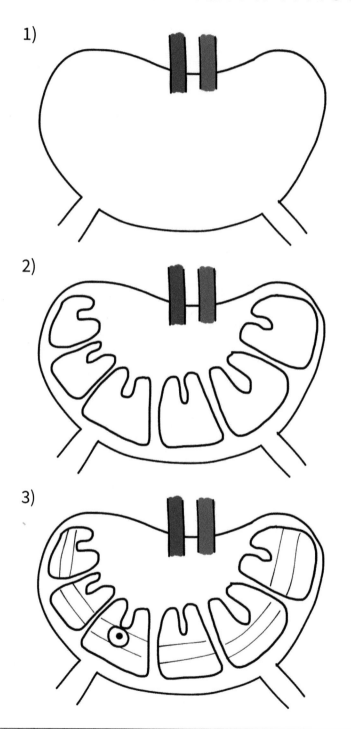

A LYMPH NODE

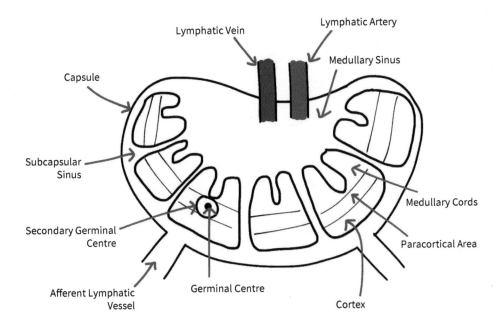

Lymphatic Vein

Lymphatic Artery

Medullary Sinus

Capsule

Subcapsular Sinus

Medullary Cords

Secondary Germinal Centre

Paracortical Area

Afferent Lymphatic Vessel

Germinal Centre

Cortex

HOW TO ... DRAW THE ARTERY HISTOLOGY

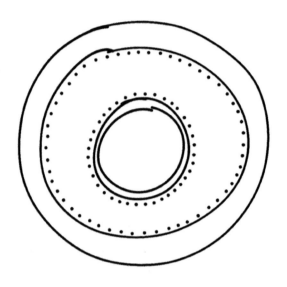

THE ARTERY HISTOLOGY

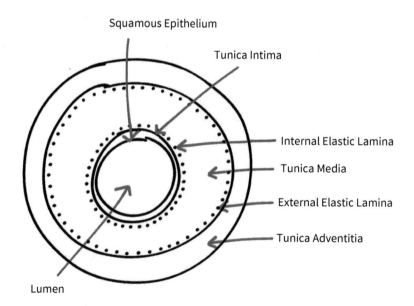

Squamous Epithelium

Tunica Intima

Internal Elastic Lamina

Tunica Media

External Elastic Lamina

Tunica Adventitia

Lumen

HOW TO ... DRAW THE VEIN HISTOLOGY

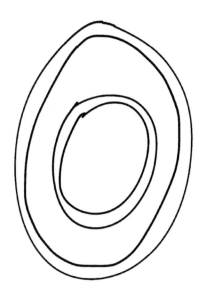

THE VEIN HISTOLOGY

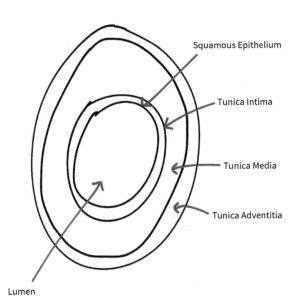

Squamous Epithelium

Tunica Intima

Tunica Media

Tunica Adventitia

Lumen

INDEX